SCIENTIFIC ASPECTS OF ACUPUNCTURE

By the same author and publisher

1 SCIENTIFIC ASPECTS OF ACUPUNCTURE (this book)
2 ACUPUNCTURE: THE ANCIENT CHINESE ART OF HEALING
3 THE MERIDIANS OF ACUPUNCTURE
4 THE TREATMENT OF DISEASE BY ACUPUNCTURE
5 ATLAS OF ACUPUNCTURE
6 ACUPUNCTURE: CURE OF MANY DISEASES

Book 1 is written for doctors. It is an attempt to explain acupuncture in terms of science.

Books 2 to 5 explain acupuncture in the traditional Chinese manner and are suitable for doctors and others interested in Far Eastern philosophy and medicine. Book 2 is a general introduction, whilst books 3 to 5 describe specific aspects.

Books 1 to 5 taken together, constitute a Textbook of Acupuncture.

Book 6 is for the non-medical reader, who wants a grasp of the essentials of acupuncture in a few hours.

SCIENTIFIC ASPECTS
OF ACUPUNCTURE

FELIX MANN

MB, BChir (Cambridge)
LMCC

Founder of The Medical Acupuncture Society

Second Edition

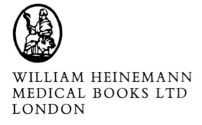

WILLIAM HEINEMANN
MEDICAL BOOKS LTD
LONDON

First published 1977
Second Edition 1983

First Edition published in Japan
by Ishiyaku in 1982

ISBN 0-433-20311-0

Printed and bound in Great Britain by
Redwood Burn Ltd, Trowbridge, Wiltshire.

CONTENTS

PREFACE to the First Edition   vii

PREFACE to the Second Edition   ix

CHAPTER I   General considerations
Neural theory of the action of acupuncture   1

CHAPTER II   Needle technique   30

CHAPTER III   Scientific versus traditional acupuncture—
some conclusions   34

CHAPTER IV   Strong reactors   41

CHAPTER V   Segmental and general sympathetic response   47

CHAPTER VI   Dermatomes, myotomes, sclerotomes   50

CHAPTER VII   Some philosophical considerations   74

CHAPTER VIII   Failed research   80

CHAPTER IX   Radiation and referred sensation of pain   89

CHAPTER X   Reflexes elicited by strong stimulation   92

CHAPTER XI   Diffuse noxious inhibitory control
by Anthony Dickenson   94

CHAPTER XII   Acupuncture analgesia: an elusive enigma   98

PREFACE TO THE FIRST EDITION

This book is an *attempt* to explain certain aspects of acupuncture in terms of science. It is not a scientific textbook of acupuncture, for at the moment I do not think it possible to write one.

The first three chapters are largely taken from the three scientific chapters of the 2nd edition of my *Acupuncture: The Ancient Chinese Art of Healing* (which will not contain these three chapters in its 3rd edition). I have included recent research, which describes in greater detail the original ideas expressed in these three chapters. The remainder of this book consists of entirely new material.

My other four books (apart from my popular book) have thus become, to a greater or lesser extent, a four volume textbook of the traditional type of acupuncture. The traditional textbook should really be read at the same time as this more scientific volume in order to be able to appreciate the subject. Some sections of these traditional books are based on modern observations: e.g. the description of periosteal acupuncture.

Recently, research into acupuncture and related subjects has increased, and may be read in a large number of journals. Perhaps not surprisingly it contains many contradictions, which do not necessarily agree with the clinician's experience. This slim book, as the title implies, discusses only certain aspects.

At a later date I hope to expand *Scientific Aspects of Acupuncture*. This will depend to a large extent on other doctors' and researchers' investigations, and hence might become a multiple author type of textbook. My main task has been to initiate the neurophysiological approach to acupuncture, the essentials of which were published in the above mentioned three chapters of the 1971 edition of *Acupuncture: The Ancient Chinese Art of Healing*. I will be glad if my investigations have sown a seed that others may tend further.

In this book I have quoted extensively from the research of others. My friends and colleagues have helped considerably by drawing my attention to articles which they thought would help my neurophysiological investigations of acupuncture, and by sending me relevant reprints. Amongst these have been David Sinclair, professor of Anatomy at Aberdeen; John Bakody, neurosurgeon of Iowa; Gerald Looney, Lecturer at U.C.L.A.; Ken Lingingston, neurosurgeon of Toronto . . . but these are just a few from a list of names which could go on for one or two pages.

The papers I have quoted contain research which in many instances has been repeated by a large number of different teams, though usually differing in certain details. On some occasions I could have quoted from ten similar papers, leaving me the somewhat arbitrary choice of mentioning one.

As a clinician, I have on the whole only quoted papers which fit in with my everyday clinical experience. It is therefore my patients whom I primarily thank.

My former teachers of acupuncture, the Chinese language and related subjects are mentioned in the Preface or Acknowledgements of my other books. Mrs. Francis Hickson helped the readability of the major portion of this book. Miss Sylvia Treadgold has, as in most of my other books, made the drawings.

Finally, I wish to thank the publishers, especially Mr. Richard Emery, and Miss Ninetta Martyn.

Doctors who wish to study acupuncture are welcome to write to me. From time to time I give courses, largely of a practical nature, during which I concentrate on those aspects of the subject that are difficult to describe in a book. These courses are only open to fully qualified and registered doctors, who have practiced orthodox medicine for at least one year, as the way in which I practice acupuncture requires just as great a knowledge of orthodox medicine as that required by a doctor practicing Western medicine.

FELIX MANN

LONDON, W.I. 1977

PREFACE TO THE SECOND EDITION

Five short new chapters (and Macdonald's research in Chapter VII), have been added to the original seven chapters. These seven chapters were in turn an expansion of three chapters of one of my earlier books.

The original three chapters still contain a few traditional concepts which have been largely superseded in the newer chapters.

I must thank mainly other doctors whose lectures I have heard, papers I have read, or who have sent me relevant references to read.

Chapter XI by Anthony Dickenson, describes research performed by him and his colleagues. Possibly this volume will gradually evolve, in future editions, into a multiple author type of book.

Those of us who practice or conduct research into acupuncture, are painfully aware of the endless contradictions which arise. I hope this book sheds light on a few of them.

I have not mentioned the endogenous opiods, as I cannot determine their importance in therapeutic acupuncture, though possibly they play a greater role in acupuncture analgesia.

LONDON W. I. 1983   FELIX MANN

I

GENERAL CONSIDERATIONS

When I first studied acupuncture in 1958, I did so in the traditional Chinese manner. A scientific approach to acupuncture hardly existed at that time. Thus I trod the pathway of Yin and Yang, the five elements, and the other accoutrements of this effective, yet fairy-tale world. I even spent ten years learning to read medical Chinese, so as to be able to read with my Chinese teacher the ancient and modern books in their original language; and what is more to be able to soak myself in the mentality and thought of this traditional medical art.

After some years, I felt I had to a certain extent mastered the subject: I knew what the ancients said, and also what was preached in this century in the East and the West. It was only then that I seriously examined the validity of all I had learnt, only to discover that most of it was phantasy,

In this book I will show that acupuncture points do not exist, meridians do not exist, and that most of the laws of acupuncture are laws about non-existent entities.

Yet acupuncture works; indeed I practise it nearly 100 per cent of my time. I hope in the ensuing pages to explain, at least partially, how acupuncture works from a neurophysiological point of view, and hence how a Western doctor may practise acupuncture and, as a corollary, why the ancients had good results by acupuncture for the wrong reasons.

I will show that an acupuncture point is like McBurney's point which can vary in size and position to a considerable extent. When the appendicitis is cured, McBurney's point disappears. The reflex

pain one has in lumbago or sciatica similar to the pain in the neck,
shoulder and arm in cervical disease would in traditional Chinese
terms be explained as the pain in an acupuncture point (if only a
small area is painful) or as the pain along a meridian (in sciatica or
brachial neuralgia).

Clearly it is more appropriate for a scientific doctor to say there
is a reflex tenderness in the renal angle in renal disease, than for him
to say there is an acupuncture point there. Likewise one should
describe the tenderness of the arm in angina pectoris as a reflex rather
than as a meridian.

In this book, I not infrequently mention acupuncture points and
meridians, even though they have no physical reality. I do this so
that those doctors who already know acupuncture may more easily
integrate tradition with the scientific.

NEURAL THEORY OF THE ACTION
OF ACUPUNCTURE

In acupuncture, the needle is frequently placed at the opposite end,
and possibly opposite side, of the body from that of the diseased
organ or site of symptoms. Under certain conditions one of these
distant and contralateral pricks can have an effect in one or two
seconds. This speed of conduction excludes the blood and lymphatic
systems (at least in this type of response) and leaves to my way of
thinking, the nervous system as the only contender.

There are other, though non-neural, theories:

Kim Bong Han* described a special conducting system of Bong
Han ducts and corpuscles, corresponding to the course of acupuncture meridians. Kellner† has shown that some of the above theory
is based on artefacts occurring in the preparation of histological
slides. Some have thought that the meridians look like the lines of
force round a magnet and postulate a magnetic theory. Others
somehow manage to bring in quantum mechanics. A Japanese researcher thinks that there is a contraction wave following the course
of meridians, along the surface of the skeletal muscles. Some liken

---

* Kim Bong Han. On the kyungrak system. 1964, Foreign languages publishing
house, Pyongyang.

† International acupuncture conference in Vienna and German acupuncture
conference in Wiesbaden.

the pinprick in the body to the electrical discharge of a condenser. A few say the pinprick releases cortisone or histamine or adrenaline but fail to explain the specific action of the acupuncture points. I once had a theory concerning the lateral line system in fish, *which I have since discarded. I am now fairly convinced that the nervous system is the transmission system used in acupuncture. The remainder of this chapter discusses this neural acupuncture theory: part is based on well-known anatomy and physiology, part is conjecture, and part requires experimental proof.

Cutaneo-Visceral Reflex

Acupuncture is based on the fact that stimulating the skin has an effect on the internal organs and on other parts of the body, a relatively simple reflex whose therapeutic application is largely ignored in the West. Various experiments demonstrate the existence of this cutaneo-visceral reflex:

Kuntz, Haselwood; Kuntz; Richins, Brizzee†, in several series of experiments stimulated the skin on the back of rabbits or rats and found changes in the duodenum or other parts of the intestinal tract corresponding to the dermatome stimulated.

By employing a quick freeze-drying technique, it was shown that when a cold beaker of ice was applied to the back in the lower thoracic region, the arterioles in the subserosa and submucosa of the duodenum were constricted and the capillary beds in the villi were ischaemic. The vascular changes in the subserosa could also be observed *in vivo* photographically and by plethysmographic recording.

Reflex responses of the gastric musculature and the pyloric

---

* See chapter XII of the 1st edition of *Acupuncture: The Ancient Chinese Art of Healing*.

† Kuntz, A., and Haselwood, L. A. Circulatory reactions in the gastro-intestinal tract elicited by local cutaneous stimulation. American Heart Journal, 1940, 20: 743–749.

Kuntz, A. Anatomic and physiologic properties of cutaneo-visceral vasomotor reflex arcs. Journal of Neurophysiology, 1945, 8: 421–429.

Richins, C. A., and Brizzee, K. Effect of localized cutaneous stimulation on circulation in duodenal arterioles and capillary beds. Journal of Neurophysiology, 1949, 12: 131–136.

sphincter in man have been described by Freude and Ruhmann*
using a fluoroscope by means of warm, cold, chemical or mechanical
stimulation of the skin of the epigastrium. They also produced
hyperaemia of the ascending colon after it had been exposed at
operation, by applying heat to the skin of the lower abdominal wall.

Nine patients with angina pectoris or acute myocardial infarction
were investigated by Travell and Rinzler.† They found that if the
trigger areas on the front of the chest were infiltrated with procaine
or cooled with ethyl chloride, complete and prolonged relief of pain
usually ensued.

Of the first series of experiments mentioned above using rats and
rabbits, some were performed on animals with an intact nervous
system under general anaesthesia, while others were performed on
animals where the spinal cord had been transected in the lower
cervical region. There was no difference in the two types of experiment, suggesting that the cutaneo-visceral reflex is mediated on a
segmental and intersegmental level and not influenced suprasegmen-
tally.

Wernøe‡ has made similar experiments on fishes and amphibians.
In the pithed eel (with its segmental structure), stimulation of 1 sq.
cm. of skin with silver nitrate caused, after a delay of two minutes,
vasoconstriction of the (from the dermatome point of view) appropriate part of the intestine, followed by a concentric contraction
of the intestinal segment, and finally peristalsis, after which bowel
movements ceased. If a more proximal or distal part of the skin was
stimulated the corresponding sharply defined part of the gut
showed the above cycle of events. In the cod electrical stimulation of
the skin just distal to the pectoral girdle caused ischaemia of the

---

* Freude, E., and Ruhmann, W. Das thermoreflektorische Verhalten von Tonus
and Kinetik am Magen. Zeitschrift für die gesamte experimentelle Medizin, 1926,
52: 338.
   Ruhmann, W., Viscerale Schmerzlinderung durch Wärme als Segment-reflex.
Zeitschrift für die gesamte experimentelle Medizin, 1927, 57: 740.
   Ruhmann, W. Ortliche Hautreizbehandlung des Magens und Ihre physiologis-
chen Grundlagen. Archiv für Verdaungskrankheiten, 1927, 41: 336.
   † Travell, J., and Rinzler, S. H. Relief of cardiac pain by local block of somatic
trigger areas. Proceedings of the Society for Experimental Biology and Medicine,
1946, 63: 480–482.
   ‡ Wernøe, T. B. Viscero-cutane Reflexe. Pflügers Archiv für die Gesamte
Physiologie, 1925, 210: 1–34.

stomach, whilst stimulation of the skin 5 cm. distal produced ischaemia in a section of the intestine.

Three eels were taken and their brains destroyed. In addition, in the first the entire spinal cord was destroyed, in the second the distal half was destroyed and in the third the spinal cord was left intact. All the skin of the three eels was stimulated with silver nitrate. After a latent period of 2 to 4 minutes the intestine of the first eel showed vasoconstriction, that of the third eel vasodilation, while the second showed vasodilation in the proximal half and vasoconstriction in the distal half. That is: in those sections where the spinal cord is intact there was vasodilation, while in those where it was destroyed, vasoconstriction. In another eel the spinal cord was divided into several segments, of which alternating segments of the spinal cord were destroyed. On stimulating all the skin with silver nitrate, it was again found that the segments with an intact spinal cord had vasodilation whilst the others had vasoconstriction.

From the above Wernøe deduced that the vasodilation was mediated by a spinal reflex, whilst the vasoconstriction by a post-ganglionic sympathetic reflex.

Sato, Sato, Shimada and Torigata* have investigated in greater detail the cutaneo-visceral reflex:

The experiments were performed on rats: some had an intact CNS but were anaesthetized, others were decerebrate and non-anaesthetized, and yet others were spinal preparations with the cord divided at C2 and non-anaesthetized. A small water filled balloon was inserted into the pyloric area of the stomach and alterations of pressure recorded. A sympathetic postganglionic nerve branch coming from the coeliac ganglion and going to the stomach, and likewise a vagal nerve branch going to the stomach were both dissected under a binocular microscope, attached to electrodes and their discharge activities recorded.

Stimulation of the abdominal wall along either the left or right mammary line reduced the pyloric pressure, more or less equally in all three types of preparation (see Fig. 1). In the intact animal the blood pressure was slightly depressed, whilst with the decerebrate and spinal animals it was slightly raised, showing that this is not an

* Sato, A., Sato, Y., Shimada, F., Torigata, Y. Changes in gastric motility produced by nociceptive stimulation of the skin in rats. Brain Research, 1975, 87: 151–159.

important factor. Likewise adrenalectomy left the results unaltered. The inhibitory pyloric response though was completely abolished by destroying the spinal cord between T5 and T11.

Transection of both vagi in the neck did not influence the cutaneo-gastric reflex. On the other hand dividing both splanchinic nerves or crushing both coeliac ganglia abolished the reflex (see Fig. 2).

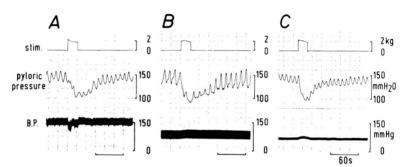

FIG. 1 A is CNS intact rat, B decerebrate, C spinal. Abdominal skin pinched with a pressure of about 2 kg. for 20 seconds. Pyloric pressure from 100–150 mm H$_2$O and 5–6 contractions per minute.

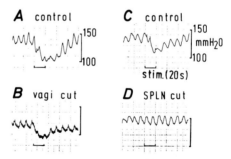

FIG. 2 A B C D rats with intact CNS. A and C control. B vagi cut. D splanchnics cut.

It was shown that when the abdominal skin was stimulated there was increased activity in the sympathetic splanchnic fibres in the CNS intact animals and also in the spinal animals, whilst there was no alteration in the recording from the vagus (see Fig. 3).

The skin of the rats was stimulated from the cervical area to the groin (see 1 to 7 in Fig. 4) along the mammary line and its extensions, in both CNS intact and spinal rats. It was found that cervical and upper thoracic stimulation had little or no depressor effect on gastric tone (1, 2 and 3), whilst upper and lower abdominal stimulation had the full effect (4, 5, 6, 7). Various other investigators have found that the cutaneo-gastric reflex is also influenced by stimulating the sciatic and femoral nerves.*

Thus it seems that this gastric inhibitory reflex is initiated by stimulating the appropriate spinal segment or any segment below it. In all these experiments of Sato *et al.* the increased sympathetic activity was observed about 1 second after stimulating the skin, whilst the reduced pyloric pressure required some 2 seconds. The maximum response was reached in about 20 seconds (hence 20 seconds was adopted as the standard time for stimulating the skin).

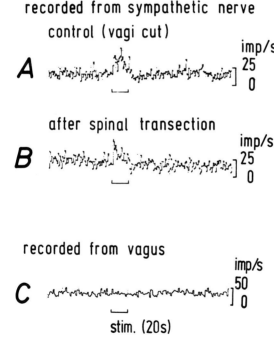

recorded from sympathetic nerve
control (vagi cut)

imp/s

A 25
0

after spinal transection

imp/s

B 25
0

recorded from vagus

imp/s

C 50
0

stim. (20s)

FIG. 3 *A* and *B* recording of gastric sympathetic nerve branch with vagi divided. *B* spinal transection also. *C* recording from vagus

* Babkin, B. P., and Kite, W. R. Jr. Central and reflex regulation of motility of pyloric antrum. Journal of Neurophysiology, 1950, 13: 321–334.

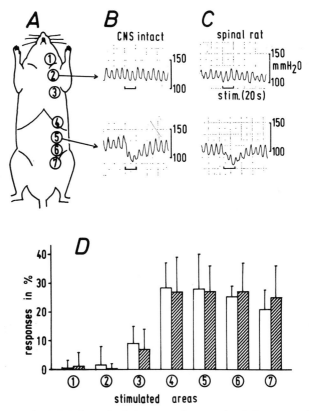

FIG. 4 Upper tracing in *B* is from stimulation area 2, lower tracing *B* from area 5. In *D* the white area represents CNS intact rats, the hatched area spinal rats

This fits in with some, but not all, of the responses one sees clinically in man.

Sato and colleagues* also investigated the reflex effect on the bladder of stimulating the skin of the perineum.

In rats the vesical pressure was kept at 40 mm H_2O. At this pressure there are small, rhythmic vesical contractions, which also occur in a denervated bladder. When the skin of the perineum was stroked or pinched, the intravesical pressure was doubled. Stimulation of the skin of the abdomen or chest had no effect. This reflex

* Sato, A., Sato, Y., Shimada, F., and Torigata, Y. Changes in vesical function produced by cutaneous stimulation in rats. Brain Research, 1975, 94: 465-474.

was observed in CNS intact animals which were anaesthetized, in decerebrate non-anaesthetized animals, and also in animals where the spinal cord had been divided in the upper cervical or mid-thoracic region. The reflex was abolished by destroying the sacral cord or by dividing the pelvic nerve branches to the bladder, which are parasympathetic. Dividing the vesical branches of the hypo-gastric nerves, which are sympathetic, had either no effect or a small equivocal effect. Direct recording of the vesical branches of the pelvic nerve, showed that whenever the perineal skin was irritated there was increased efferent discharge activity.

When the vesical pressure was instead raised to some 200 mm H_2O by injecting more water into an intravesical balloon, the vesical contractions became stronger but less frequent—micturition con-tractions. These contractions were inhibited by pinching the perin-eum, but not by pinching the abdomen or chest. This reflex occurred in animals with an intact CNS who were anaesthetized, and also in decerebrate or spinal unanaesthetized animals. The reflex was abolished if the vesical branches of the pelvic nerve were divided. Recording of the activity of the vesical branches of the pelvic nerve, showed an increase concomitant with the increase in vesical pressure during a micturition contraction.

A reflex between the abdominal skin and the duodenum has also been described by Sato and Terui*, using similar experimental methods to those used in his previous experiments.

The small rhythmic (40 per minute) waves, which correspond to the pendular movements of the duodenum, were inhibited by pinching the abdominal skin. The reflex remained intact in spinal preparations if the vagi were divided. The reflex was abolished if the splanchnics were divided.

The duodenum has also slow waves, corresponding to peristalisis (0.5 per minute). These are likewise inhibited by pinching the abdominal skin. This reflex, as that of the small waves is abolished when the splanchnics are divided.

Pastinszky, Kenedi and Fáber† have shown that stimulation of

---

* Sato, Y., Terui, N. Changes in duodenal motility produced by noxious mechanical stimulation of the skin in rats. Neuroscience Letters, 1976, 2: 189–193.

† Pastinszky, I., Kenedi, J., Fáber, U. Experimental studies of the dermato-cardiac reflex effect. Acta Physiologica Academiae Scientiarum Hungariae, 1964, 25: 89–95.

the chest wall in cats produced temporary or even permanent changes in the heart and lungs.

They shaved the left chest wall of cats, which was then painted daily with a strong irritant solution. This produced erythema and oedema of the skin and subcutaneous tissues, which often progressed to ulceration and partial microscopic necrosis. It is thus apparent that this stimulation which was applied for some four weeks, is stronger and more continuous than that in most of the experiments cited in this chapter.

The majority of the cats show E.C.G. changes such as negative T waves, partial atrio-ventricular block, sinus bradycardia, accessory rhythm, complete atrio-ventricular block or bundle branch block. Many of the cats had punctate haemorrhages of the pericardium, likewise of the lungs and pleura bilaterally. Histologically the cardiac muscle showed capillary dilation and likewise dilation of the major branches of the coronary arteries and veins. A few fibres of the cardiac muscle showed micronecrosis with disappearance of the transverse strictions.

In those cats where the skin reaction to painting with the irritant was mild, the E.C.G. changes mentioned above were likewise of a milder nature or temporary. If the skin was painted only once, a smaller proportion of cats developed E.C.G. changes, which were then of only a very temporary nature. If the right buttock instead of the left chest wall was painted, there were no E.C.G. changes whatsoever, except possibly in one equivocal case.

Viscero-Cutaneous Reflex

The cutaneo-visceral reflex mentioned in the preceding section is of prime importance in acupuncture, for it is by its mediation that an acupuncture needle placed in the correct part of the skin is able to affect the appropriate organ or diseased part of the body.

The viscero-cutaneous reflex to be discussed in this section is of importance (1) in diagnosis and (2) in lowering the threshold of stimulation required in treatment by acupuncture.

It is often noticed clinically that a disease of an internal organ will produce in some part of the skin (not infrequently of the same dermatome) pain, tenderness, hyperaesthesia, hypoaesthesia etc. This can also be seen experimentally:

Wernøe stimulated the rectum of a decapitated plaice electrically, or with copper sulphate or barium chloride. In each case the skin became pale, due to retraction of the melanophores, extending to 3 or 4 spinal segments of the appropriate dermatomes. Likewise in the eel and cod, the stomach, intestines, gall bladder or spleen were stimulated mechanically or by the intramural injection of 10 per cent adrenalin; in each case the skin becoming lighter over an area of several segments, again in the expected dermatomes.

In the decapitated cod, if the spinal cord is in addition destroyed, the viscero-cutaneous reflex is not abolished. If, on the other hand, the cord is intact but the sympathetic chain is excised the reflex is abolished. This suggests that it is not a spinal reflex, but that it is mediated along unknown paths of the sympathetic chain.

The viscero-cutaneous reflex discussed here and the viscero-motor reflex to be discussed later are presumably the mechanism whereby diseases of internal organs produce pain or tenderness of certain acupuncture points, areas of skin, or muscle spasm. Presumably other, though similar reflexes are involved when diseases other than those of internal organs likewise cause pain, tenderness, muscle spasm etc.

In acupuncture a somewhat smaller stimulus is needed if the acupuncture needle is put directly into one of these tender or painful areas or into a meridian that crosses or is related in some other way to the tender area. Presumably facilitation is taking place. This facilitation is also a safeguard, for if the acupuncture needle is put in the wrong place it has little effect, as it is easier to affect a diseased or disease related area than a healthy one.

Viscero-Motor and Viscero-Visceral Reflexes

These reflexes are in many instances similar to the viscero-cutaneous reflexes mentioned above, occurring mostly at the same time, though requiring an intact spinal cord.

Miller, Simpson* and many others stimulated the viscera and obtained muscle contractions in the expected appropriate dermatomes (and distant dermatomes—see later). Distension of the stomach by air, traction on the stomach, mustard oil on the gastric mucosa, squeezing the small intestine, mechanical stimulation of the kidney

* Miller, F. R., and Simpson, H. M. Transactions of the Royal Society of Canada, sec V, 1924, XVIII, 147.

or spleen all elicited the reflex, which could be abolished by dividing the appropriate dorsal root. The reflex from the stomach was stopped by dividing the splanchnic nerves, while stimulation of the central ends of the divided nerve restored it; similar results were obtained with the superior mesenteric nerves for the small intestine, the hypogastric nerve for the kidney, and the splenic nerve for the spleen.

Brown-Sequard* relates an experiment with a dog which had a tube tied into its ureter. When the internal abdominal wall was pricked within the distribution of the 1st lumbar nerve, the secretion of urine was considerably diminished.

Brown-Sequard* also quotes the case of a colleague, Sir Benjamin Brodie, who had a patient with a stricture of the urethra causing pain and lameness of the foot. All symptoms were relieved after a bougie had been passed up the urethra. The urethra and foot symptoms were probably in the same or neighbouring dermatome. I have on several occasions observed in a patient with multiple sclerosis that when the heel is pricked with a needle the patient micturates.

Cannon and Murphy† compared two series of cats who had been given ether anaesthesia. The one group had their testicles crushed whilst the others were not molested. Afterwards both groups were given food mixed with barium and its passage in the ileum followed roentgenologically. In the emasculated group there was no movement of the ileum for 4 hours, after which it started sluggishly; whilst in the control group there was movement from the very beginning. The testicles are usually given as T10 to L3 (varying according to the author) and the small intestine as T6 to T11, so that this is possibly a segmental reflex.

Dermatomes and Acupuncture Points

Some of the acupuncture points, particularly those on the back, having an effect on a specific organ, are in the appropriate dermatomes as a glance at Fig. 5‡ and 6 will show. Account should be

* Brown-Sequard, C. E., Course of lectures on the physiology and pathology of the central nervous system. 1860, Lippincott, Philadelphia, p. 170 and 167.

† Cannon, W. B., and Murphy, F. T. Physiologic Observations in experimentally produced ileus. Journal of the American Medical Association, 1907, 49: 840.

‡ Dermatomes derived from Hansen, K. and Schliak, H. Segmentale innervation, ihre bedeutung für Klinik und Praxis, 1962, Georg Thieme, Stuttgart; and other sources.

taken though that the Chinese do not always mean the same as we
do when they say heart, liver, etc. as described in greater detail in
'The Meridians of Acupuncture'.

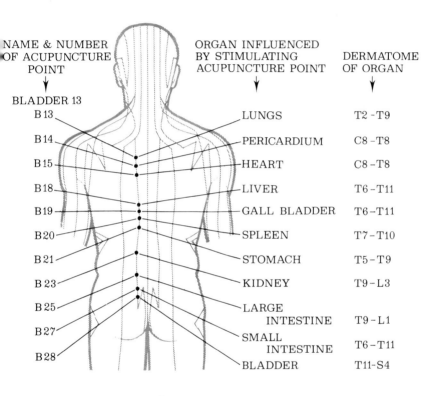

NAME & NUMBER OF ACUPUNCTURE POINT	ORGAN INFLUENCED BY STIMULATING ACUPUNCTURE POINT	DERMATOME OF ORGAN
BLADDER 13		
B 13	LUNGS	T2 - T9
B 14	PERICARDIUM	C8 - T8
B 15	HEART	C8 - T8
B 18	LIVER	T6 - T11
B 19	GALL BLADDER	T6 - T11
B 20	SPLEEN	T7 - T10
B 21	STOMACH	T5 - T9
B 23	KIDNEY	T9 - L3
B 25	LARGE INTESTINE	T9 - L1
B 27	SMALL INTESTINE	T6 - T11
B 28	BLADDER	T11-S4

FIG. 5 Hyperaesthetic zones in internal disease

The majority of reflexes mentioned in the previous section
(cutaneo-visceral, viscero-cutaneous, viscero-motor) are segmental in
nature, and hence fit in with the dermatome pattern of acupuncture
points described in this section. Some of the reflexes can also be
intersegmental, not following the dermatomes. These are described
in the next section.

There is often considerable variation in the dermatome pattern
according to the method of investigation: hyposensitivity from loss

of function of a single nerve root (Keegan and Garrett);* electrical skin resistance in sympathectomised patients; electrical skin resistance on stimulation of anterior spinal roots; pain distribution after hypertonic saline injection of interspinous ligaments (Kellgren).

There is also variation between individuals: Sixteen patients were examined to determine the electrical skin resistance of the arm at operation,† by stimulating the anterior spinal roots. The upper limit

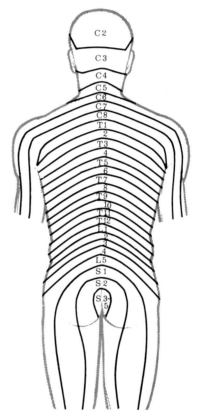

FIG. 6 Dermatomes, after Keegan and Garrett

* Keegan, J. J., and Garrett, F. D. The segmental distribution of the cutaneous nerves in the limbs of man. Anatomical Record, 1948, 102: 409–439. Also Fig. 6.

† Ray, B. S., Hinsey, J. C., Geohegan, W. A. Observations on the distribution of the sympathetic nerves to the pupil and upper extremity as determined by stimulation of the anterior roots in man. Annals of Surgery, 1943, 118, No. 4: 647–655.

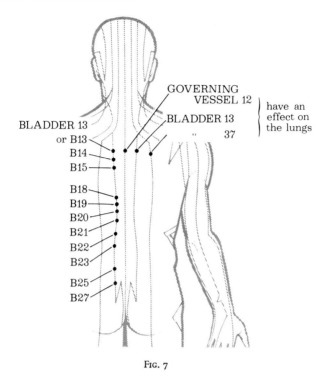

FIG. 7

varied from T1 to T3, whilst the lower limit varied from T7 to T10. The usual range is T2 to T9.

Normally the dermatome of the arm is given as C5 to T1, whilst the sympathetic dermatome obtained by stimulating the anterior spinal root is T2 to T9. When the skin and deeper tissues are pierced by an acupuncture needle both the spinal nerves and the sympathetic nerves of the blood vessels are affected, that of the sympathetic nerves having no effect unless one believes in antidromic stimulation, or as more recently in autonomic afferents.

The series of acupuncture points on the black lateral to the associated points shown in Fig. 7 have an effect on the same organ as its sister point at the same level, e.g. both B13 and B37 influence the lungs (likewise the points on the governing vessel).

The abdomen and front of the chest are traversed by the spleen, stomach, kidney and conception meridians (Fig. 8), which despite their names have, I find, an effect mainly on the region of the body

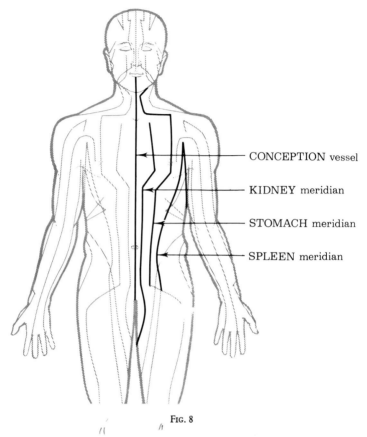

CONCEPTION vessel

KIDNEY meridian

STOMACH meridian

SPLEEN meridian

Fig. 8

traversed. All four meridians where they cross the chest may be used to treat the lungs and heart, yet their abdominal course influences the abdominal viscera. Thus as with the acupuncture points on the back a rough dermatomal pattern is preserved.

It is interesting to note that the majority of acupuncture points on the abdomen, thorax and back are near the mid-ventral and mid-dorsal lines. This corresponds to the segmental reference of deep pain obtained by Kellgren* when injecting hypertonic saline into the interspinous ligaments (Fig. 9).

* Kellgren, J. H. On the distribution of pain arising from deep somatic structures with charts of segmental pain. Clinical Science, 1939–42, 4: 35–46. Also Fig. 9.

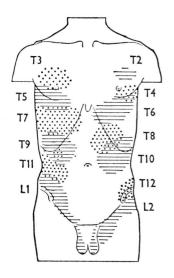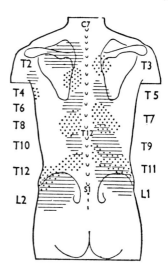

FIG. 9

The meridians of the lung, pericardium and heart on the anterior surface of the arm correspond at least approximately to the appropriate dermatome (Fig. 10). The meridians on the posterior surface of the arm: the large intestine, small intestine and triple warmer, do not correspond to the appropriate dermatome (Fig. 11).

In actual practice the situation is somewhat different, even for those meridians that follow a roughly dermatomal pattern.

If a patient has angina pectoris he may have pain or tenderness in the region of the heart meridian on the medial side of the arm. Just as frequently he may have pain or tenderness in the region of the lung meridian on the lateral side of the arm. Indeed the pain may appear in any part of the arm, along the course of (or in between) any of the six meridians of the arm, or even in the chest, neck or jaw.

Thus clearly the heart meridian cannot exist. It would be true though to say that pain from the heart, pericardium and lung, may be in the arm (and elsewhere), but the essential is that it may be *anywhere in the arm*.

In this section we have discussed the acupuncture points that more or less fit in with a dermatological pattern (Fig. 12),* namely—the

* From Ranson, S. W. and Clark, S. L. The anatomy of the nervous system, 1966, Saunders, Philadelphia.

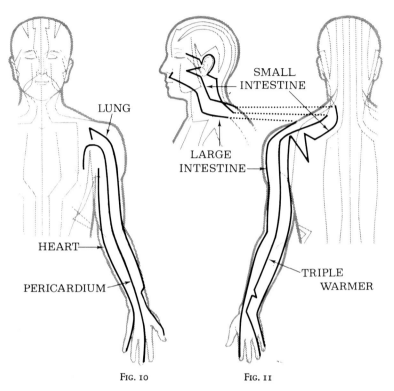

LUNG

SMALL
INTESTINE

LARGE
INTESTINE

HEART

PERICARDIUM

TRIPLE
WARMER

FIG. 10   FIG. 11

whole of the back, the abdomen, the front of the chest and the arms. The acupuncture points of the legs and head do not fit in with what is known of dermatomes and are therefore described in relation to other neurological concepts below:

Intersegmental Reflexes and Acupuncture Points

The acupuncture points on the legs are those of the liver, gall bladder, kidney, bladder, spleen and stomach. In all cases (except the bladder) the dermatomes of these organs are on the trunk and not on the legs. It is however an undoubted fact, observed every day by any doctor who practises acupuncture (for the leg acupuncture points are commonly used), that stimulation of a leg acupuncture point does have an effect on the appropriate organ, even though it may be ten dermatomes away. A possible explanation is via intersegmental

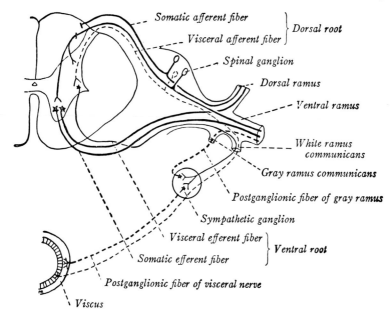

Somatic afferent fiber
Visceral afferent fiber } Dorsal **root**
Spinal ganglion
Dorsal ramus
Ventral **ramus**
White ramus communicans
Gray ramus communicans
Postganglionic fiber of gray **ramus**
Sympathetic ganglion
Visceral efferent fiber }
Somatic efferent fiber } Ventral **root**
Postganglionic fiber of visceral nerve
Viscus

FIG. 12 The peripheral nerves and spinal cord

reflexes, called by Sherrington long reflexes, whilst those effects of acupuncture that fit in with the dermatomes are segmental reflexes—Sherrington's short reflexes.

Sherrington* described the *scratch reflex* in the spinal dog (Fig. 13) in which stimulation anywhere in a saddle-shaped area extending from the pectoral to the pelvic girdle caused rapid scratching movements in the ipselateral hind leg and rigidity in the contralateral limb. If the stimulus is moved but slightly to the opposite side of the back the hind legs reverse their roles. Ipsilateral hemisection of the spinal cord abolishes the reflex, contralateral hemisection leaves it unaffected.

Sherrington also experimented with decerebrate cats in which the nervous axis is divided at the level of the mid-brain. In the resultant decerebrate rigidity, the cats exhibit *reflex figures* (Fig. 14).

(*a*) In normal decerebrate rigidity all limbs are extended.

* Sherrington, C. S. The integrative action of the nervous system, 1906, Scribner, New York. Also Fig. 13 and 14.

(*b*) If the left pinna is stimulated there is flexion of the left fore and right hind limbs, with increased extension of the others.

(*c*) If the left fore limb is stimulated there is flexion of the left fore and right hind limbs, with increased extension of the others.

(*d*) If the left hind limb is stimulated there is flexion of the left hind limb and right fore limb, with increased extension of the others.

The reflex figures require both sides of the spinal cord for their conduction, not only the one as in the scratch reflex. Both the scratch reflex and reflex figures are intersegmental (jumping several dermatomes) cutaneo-motor reflexes.

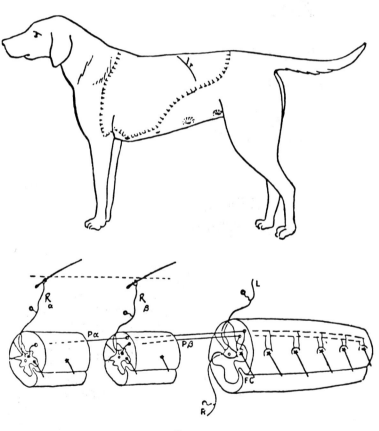

FIG. 13

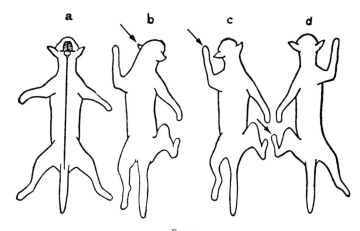

FIG. 14

Downman* investigated long viscero-motor and long cutaneo-motor reflexes in the cat with a spinal transection at T1. The splanchnic nerve serving the viscera, intercostal nerves T3-T13, lumbar nerves L1-L3 and the tibial nerve at the knee were all exteriorised.

Maximal single-shock stimulation of the central end of the splanchnic nerve evoked reflex volleys in all body wall nerves and the tibial nerve (Fig. 15). Even at threshold stimulation several intercostal nerves were involved. If an intercostal nerve was stimulated the response was in some cases as large as with splanchnic stimulation.

Downman showed that splanchnic excitation can spread up the cord by (1) a fast extraspinal route in the sympathetic chain of the same side and (2) a slower intraspinal route of limited ascent. Intercostal excitation can ascend only by a slow intraspinal route. This was demonstrated by the following experiments: Reflex discharges into the lower intercostal nerves on both sides were elicited by stimulating the left splanchnic nerve. Cutting the left sympathetic chain limited the upward spread of the excitation to the

* Downman, C. B. B. Skeletal muscle reflexes of splanchnic and intercostal nerve origin in acute spinal and decerebrate cats. Journal of Neurophysiology, 1955, 18: 217–235. Also Fig. 15.
Downman, C. B. B., and McSwiney, B. A. Reflexes elicited by visceral stimulation in the acute spinal animal. Journal of Physiology, 1946, 105: 80–94.

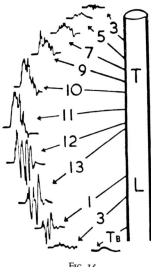

FIG. 15

next 3 to 5 segments of the cord. The discharges in the nerves were now of decreasing size and of longer latency in these segments. Spread of activity on stimulating a lower left intercostal nerve was unaffected. Where the chain had been left intact and the cord transected, splanchnic excitation spread freely into segments above the transection, but spread of intercostal excitation stopped at this level. In those instances where there is a contralateral response, experiments involving unilateral section of the dorsal nerve roots were performed. It was concluded that the splanchnic afferent volleys enter the cord by the dorsal root, traverse the spinal cord and leave by the contralateral intercostal nerves. Similar research has been done by Miller, Ward,* and Duda.†

The movements of the intercostals and tibialis anterior on stimulation of the splanchnics are considerably increased if a spinal instead of a decerebrate cat is used.

* Miller, F. R., and Ward, R. A. Viscero-motor reflexes. American Journal of Physiology, 1925, 73: 329–340.

† Duda, P. Facilitatory and inhibitory effects of splanchnic afferentation on somatic reflexes. Physiologia Bohemoslovenica, 1964, 13: 137–141.

Duda, P. Localization of the splanchnic effect on somatic reflexes in the spinal cord. Physiologia Bohemoslovenica, 1964, 13: 142–147.

Downmann and Hussain* showed that the main descending inhibitory tract is in the dorsal third of the lateral funiculus of the same side. This was demonstrated by sectioning various parts of the cord (most of which had a slight effect) and finding which had the major inhibitory influence (Fig. 16). Likewise deep cuts in the lower medulla, at the level of the middle of the cuneate tubercles, caused full release. Shen Eh† and colleagues have more recently performed similar experiments.

Harrison, Calhoun and Harrison‡ have shown that movement of the hind leg in a dog causes increased respiration—another example of an intersegmental reflex.

In their experiments, the hind leg of a dog was completely severed from the rest of the body at the hip joint, with preservation of only the sciatic nerve and femoral artery and vein. Passive movement of the hind leg produced within seconds an increased volume of

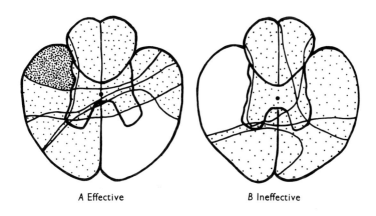

A Effective   B Ineffective

Fig. 16

* Downmann, C. B. B., Hussain, A. Spinal tracts and supraspinal centres influencing visceromotor and allied reflexes in cats. Journal of Physiology, 1958, 141: 489–499. Also Fig. 16.

† Shen Eh, Ts'ai T'i-tao, Lan Ch'ing. Supraspinal participation in the inhibitory effect of acupuncture on viscero-somatic reflex discharges. Chinese Medical Journal, 1975; 1 (6): 431–440.

‡ Harrison, W. G., Calhourn, J. A., Harrison, T. R. Afferent impulses as a cause of increased ventilation during muscular exercise. American Journal of Physiology, 1932, 100: 68–73.

respiration whether the femoral artery and vein were occluded with clamps or not. The respiration returned to normal only two minutes after movement of the leg was stopped. When the sciatic nerve was divided the reflex was abolished.

There are also long intersegmental viscero-visceral reflexes. The gastric-colic reflex is invoked when food entering the stomach causes mass contractions of the colon. Likewise in travel sickness where the afferent fibres are the trigeminal, glossopharygneal or vagus and the efferents are the phrenics and intercostal nerves.

I have thus been able to show in this section that the leg muscles contract if, under the correct conditions, one stimulates: the abdominal viscera, the splanchnics, the intercostal nerves, the outer ear, the front feet, the skin of the back in the upper thoracic region and other areas many segments away from the dermatomes of the human leg (or hind leg in animals). The reverse of the above namely stimulating the skin of the leg having an effect on the viscera, was demonstrated by Brown-Sequard in the same course of lectures mentioned earlier. He poured boiling water over the hind leg of a dog whose spine was divided at L3 and another dog whose spine was divided at T3. At autopsy two days later the former dog showed congestion of the bladder and rectum (segmental), whilst in the latter all abdominal organs were congested (intersegmental).

The distribution of the acupuncture points on the legs is such that each organ corresponds to several dermatomes and each dermatome corresponds to several organs.

There are six meridians representing six organs in the leg. The course of the meridians would suggest that treating the shin over which the stomach meridian courses, or treating the calf over which the bladder meridian courses, would be the most appropriate. As mentioned previously in connection with the arm, this is not correct. A reflexly tender area may appear in either the shin or the calf in disease of the stomach or bladder or vica versa. Indeed as with the arm, the reflex tenderness associated with the lower six organs may appear almost anywhere on the legs (and the lower abdomen and back), though in certain instances it tends to appear more often in certain areas.

Traditionally the meridians of the small and large intestines are on the arm. In my opinion this is completely wrong, as with a few exceptions, these organs can only be treated by stimulation of the lower half of the body. The triple warmer defies definition—though I have described it in my books on traditional acupuncture.

The problem is not too simple, as investigations by Travell and Bigelow* showed. In patients with pain encompassing several dermatomes it was found that a pinprick to the trigger area might relieve the pain in that dermatome or in several dermatomes or in one dermatome, then miss out a dermatome to relieve pain again in a further dermatome.

Acupuncture Points on the Head — Near and Distant Effects

Most of the acupuncture points on the head have a local effect, which could presumably be explained by local reflex arcs similar to segmental reflexes.

The apportioning of the acupuncture points on the head to the various internal organs is hard to follow both theoretically and in actual clinical acupuncture practice, though distant effects undoubtedly occur.

Koblank† investigated a reflex between the nose and the heart. He found a sharply defined area in the region of the superior concha of the nose, which if stimulated with a probe caused various cardiac arrhythmias in man, dogs and rabbits. When the vagus was cut on one side, the reflex remained intact; when cut on both sides the reflex was abolished for a few days and then returned, but weaker than formerly. When the maxillary nerve was divided on one side the reflex was permanently abolished when the same side of the nose was stimulated, but the reflex persisted normally when the healthy side was stimulated. From this it was deduced that the trigeminal nerve relayed the stimulation of the nasal mucous membrane to the region of the nucleus of the vagus, which then passed it on via the vagus to the heart. It was considered though that there was more than one final pathway as dividing the vagus only partially abolished the reflex.

Koblank also investigated the relation between the lower turbinate of the nose and the reproductive organs of rabbits and dogs. He found that if the lower turbinate was excised in young animals that

* Travell, J., and Bigelow, N. H. Referred somatic pain does not follow a simple segmental pattern. Federation Proceedings, 1946, 5: 106.
† Alfred Koblank. Die Nase als Reflexorgan. 1958. Haug. Ulm. Also Fig. 17.

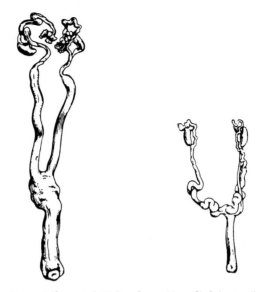

FIG. 17 Left: control. Right: after excision of inferior turnibate

the uterus, fallopian tubes, ovary or testicle failed to develop, even though the adult animal attained the same weight as an unoperated control. The failure of development showed itself both as a considerable reduction in size (Fig. 17) and histologically.

Koblank, Röder and Bickel experimented with dogs who had a Pavlov type exteriorised blind loop, whereby changes in gastric secretion and motility could be observed directly. They found that when the 'stomach area' on the anterior third of the middle turbinate was stimulated that the gastric secretion and movement were increased.

It should be noted that in the above experiments stimulation of the upper turbinate affected the heart, the middle turbinate the stomach, and the lower turbinate the reproductive organs.

Specific Response versus Generalised Response

In the practice of acupuncture it is sometimes found that one (or a small group) of acupuncture points are effective in treating a certain patient. On other occasions, any one of several meridians (encompassing a large number of acupuncture points) can be effective.

In the former case a specific stimulus is mandatory, in the latter nearly any general stimulus is all that is needed.·

The specific response presumably takes place, along the lines of the nervous pathways described in the previous sections.

The generalised hypersensitivity on the other hand seems similar to the pain one can sometimes have with severe toothache when the whole of the same side of the face, arm and upper chest are hypersensitive. In the same way the viscera may sometimes become hypersensitive affecting the nerves in a large area, and hence only require in treatment an acupuncture needle put anywhere in a large area, in any of a large number of acupuncture points, or in any of several meridians.

In other cases a stimulus anywhere in a large area does not depend on hypersensitivity, but on the large number of neurones that have a final common path. Ashkenaz* stimulated the gall bladder of cats by inflating a balloon. This caused contraction of the panniculus carnosus muscle (the cat's equivalent of the platysma, but extending over most of the body). This viscero-pannicular reflex was only abolished when all the dorsal roots T2 to T9 were severed, a single root being sufficient to preserve the reflex, thus demonstrating the convergence that can take place.

Diseased organs seem to have a lowered threshold of response, for only a small stimulus is needed to correct a dysfunction of a diseased organ. On the other hand a very considerable stimulus is needed to alter the function of a healthy organ. For this reason the small prick of an acupuncture needle can cure some of the severest diseases, and yet is normally harmless if the wrong treatment is effected, as the threshold of response of the healthy organ is beyond the stimulus of a mere needle prick.

It should be noted that the Chinese describe the acupuncture points as being quite small—a matter of millimetres. In my experience this is only true to a limited extent, for not infrequently a stimulus anywhere in an area as large as a dermatome (or several dermatomes if there has been spread of hypersensitivity) is sufficient. If this largish area is carefully examined by hand a few small areas

* Ashkenaz, D. M. An experimental analysis of centripetal visceral pathways based upon the viscero-pannicular reflex. American Journal of Physiology, 1937. 120: 587–595.

of maximal tenderness, with possibly small fibrositic-like nodules, will be found (similar to the small areas of maximal tenderness found when a large area such as the neck and shoulders are 'rheumatic'). If these small areas of maximal tenderness, or the 'fibrositic' nodules are stimulated by an acupuncture needle the response is normally greater than when the surrounding less tender area is needled. If the dysfunction of a diseased organ is mild, a reflex tenderness may not be produced over the whole of a dermatome, being demonstrable only in a few small tender areas—the same areas as mentioned a few lines above. These small tender areas of 'fibrositic' nodules are relatively constant in position, whether the remaining surrounding part of the dermatome is tender or not. This constancy in position applies from one individual to another, and is likewise the same for any variety of diseases producing a reflex tenderness in that area. It is these small tender areas of constant position, which are termed the acupuncture points; although, as mentioned above, a stimulus anywhere in the appropriate dermatome (or sometimes even larger area) may work, albeit frequently not so well. Sometimes stimulation anywhere in the correct quarter of the body is sufficient.

Some years ago David Sinclair, professor of anatomy at Aberdeen University, wrote an as yet unpublished paper, which he has kindly let me read, concerning the reflexes between the skin and viscera defined as viscero-somatic, somato-somatic, viscero-visceral, somato-visceral. In this article Sinclair quotes a hundred papers (several of which are mentioned in this chapter) concerning these reflexes which are the presumed mechanism of acupuncture—though probably most of the authors know nothing or little of acupuncture. At the time of writing and in other papers* Sinclair advanced a branched axon theory partially to explain the observed phenomena, but since then he thinks the more conventional nervous pathways are the mediator.

It is remarkable that the stimulation of the skin for a few seconds, should activate a nerve reflex in such a manner, that the dysfunction

---

* Sinclair, D. C. The remote reference of pain aroused in the skin. Brain, 1949, 72: 364.

Sinclair, D. C., Weddell, G., and Feindel, W. Referred pain and associated phenomena. Brain, 1948, 71: 184.

of the diseased area should be alleviated for a long time or even permanently.

The same phenomenon is observed when the dorsal columns of the spinal cord, or a peripheral nerve, are electrically stimulated in patients with permanent intractable pain. Before the implantation of a stimulator these patients require the *continuous* administration of analgesics. After implantation stimulation for a *short while*, will in the more responsive patients produce analgesia for half a day to one week.

In acupuncture, after the appropriate skin area has been stimulated a few times, the resultant relief of symptoms may be permanent, i.e. there is a cure. This does not happen in dorsal column or peripheral nerve stimulation, for the type of patient to whom this is normally applied has an irreversible pathological process. In acupuncture on the other hand, most patients have diseases which are physiologically reversible.

II

NEEDLE TECHNIQUE

The only thing of importance in acupuncture is to stimulate the right place. What the stimulus is, is of secondary importance.

Normally a needle is used, and this, in my experience, is the most effective. Massage, various types of electrical stimuli, mechanical vibrators, heating, magnetic oscillators have all been tried but are not quite as effective. In the Far East the pith of Artemesia Japonica (moxa) is dried and rolled into balls about two millimetres in diameter; one is placed on the acupuncture point of choice and lit so that it glows like the lighted end of a cigarette. This is an effective stimulus, but it may cause burns and even scars which do not necessarily disappear. This method, called moxibustion is supposed to be more effective in diseases due to cold and dampness, but in my experience this is not the case; and as it is no more effective than a needle I rarely use it. Another type of heating treatment, used in diseases due to cold and damp is to use the long handled type of Chinese needle. About an inch is cut off a moxa stick which is shaped like a cigar, and pushed over the exposed part of the needle. The moxa is lit and the heat is conducted down the shaft of the needle to the surrounding skin and flesh. As I find this no more effective than simple needling, I rarely use it. There are many old and modern variations to the above, but none are as simple and effective as a needle.

The needles may be made of any material. Silver alloys have the advantage of having some self-sterilising properties, which is an additional secondary safeguard. Stainless steel is best for thin needles as silver is too soft. Stainless steel needles have to be thrown away when they become blunt as they are difficult to resharpen. Silver needles can be resharpened on a very fine carborundum or other stone. The silver needles are best sharpened on several surfaces so that the tip is a cross between the cone of an ordinary sewing needle and the pyramid of a leather cutting needle. In this way they pierce the skin more easily yet do not cause bleeding as easily as a leather cutting or surgical needle. The much finer stainless steel needles should be sharpened like a cone, as is usual for ordinary needles. Injection needles may be used, but they easily cause bleeding and theoretically could harbour some dirt in the hollow of the needle; while a solid acupuncture needle, is, as it were, wiped clean on all its surfaces in its passage through the skin. If it is intended to leave the needle in place, it will be found that the head of an injection needle is rather heavy and pulls the needle out of place. I use a hot air steriliser. Small, cheap, automatic ones are sold in dental equipment shops.

Some European doctors differentiate between silver and gold needles founded on a misconception of tonification and sedation (see below). This may have arisen as a translating error as in Chinese the characters for gold and metal are the same. I have found no reference to it in the Chinese literature, though possibly it exists. Whilst in China, several doctors asked me what this new invention concerning silver and gold needles as used in Europe was all about!

Traditional Chinese works on acupuncture describe at great length about fifty different ways of inserting acupuncture needles, with names such as: 'burning mountain fire technique' or 'green dragon wagging tail technique'. These techniques involve the following: Inserting the needle 3 or 9 or 81 times; pointing the needle with or against the direction of flow of Qi along a meridian; twisting the needle clockwise or anticlockwise; inserting the needle fast and taking it out slowly as opposed to slowly in and fast out; inserting the needle in three stages and pulling it out in one as opposed to insertion in one stage and pulling out in three—and many more refinements. I have tried assiduously to find a difference between these methods, but have come to the conclusion that basically there is no difference except insofar as it includes what is said in the ensuing lines.

The size of the stimulus increases with:

1. A fat needle.
2. The deeper the insertion.
3. The more the needle is pushed up and down or twisted, so that
   the tip causes greater localised trauma.
4. A blunt needle or one with a hook on the end (both undesirable).
5. The more acupuncture points are used having a similar effect
   (sometimes has severe effect).
6. Leaving the needle in longer (extremely doubtful).
7. Repeating the treatment at frequent intervals.

Many doctors think that the bigger the stimulus, the greater the effect; but just as often it is the very reverse. I have many patients who respond best to only one or two shallow pricks with thin, sharp needles, with the needle not left in place and the treatment repeated only infrequently. Certain constitutional types respond best to light treatment, others to heavy treatment, just as certain patients respond best to small and sometimes even microscopic doses of ordinary drugs while average doses of drugs may have no effect or make them feel ill. Because I recognise this great variation in individual sensitivity I have on occasions been able to successfully treat a patient by giving them a half to a tenth of the same medicine as their general practitioner was unsuccessfully giving them. Most chronic conditions I treat only fortnightly and finish the treatment at even longer intervals, for sometimes the effect of a treatment is only apparent after a week or more and if the second treatment is done before the effect of the first one is apparent, the two treatments may antagonise one another with either no result or a temporary worsening of the patient's condition. Acute conditions may be treated more frequently. Patients whom I see from abroad I of course treat at more frequent intervals; but it requires greater clinical experience and judgement on the doctor's part.

Chinese and European acupuncturists differentiate between tonification and sedation. Diagnostically one can say certain conditions represent underactivity whilst others represent overactivity. If for example the pulse is fine and weak one says it is underactive and requires tonification; if the pulse is strong and full one says it is overactive and the appropriate organ requires sedation. The Chinese and many Europeans also say that if the needle is inserted in a certain way, or one uses a silver needle, or one uses a point of sedation, that the appropriate organ is sedated; likewise if one inserts the needle in a different way, uses a gold needle, or a point of tonification, the same organ is tonified. I find on the contrary that whatever is done, as diagnosed on the pulse, the organ is brought nearer normality. If for example the pulse in the position of the heart is overactive (pulse full and strong) then whichever needle technique one uses, whatever the needle is made from and whichever point of the heart meridian one uses, the effect is the same: namely that the pulse becomes nearer that of a fine and weak pulse. Likewise if the pulse had been underactive (pulse fine and weak) and one had done exactly the same as above, the pulse would have become stronger. In other words the needle seems to exert a normalising influence: sedating the overactive, and tonifying the underactive; and if the doctor wishes it or not, he cannot (except under a few rare conditions) do the reverse. This normalising influence could fit in with the way the autonomic nervous system functions. It is interesting, at least philosophically, that overactivity and underactivity can be diagnosed, but that the treatment does not differentiate the two. Whether or not overactivity and underactivity are important from the point of view of Chinese traditional herbal medicine I do not know. In their theory it is important but perhaps not in reality.

The above jeopardises the whole idea of polarity, of Yin and Yang, coupled organs, hot and cold diseases, full and empty diseases, tonification and sedation, the five element theory, the mother-son law, the husband-wife law, the midday-midnight law. In fact this clearly demonstrates that nearly all the traditional theoretical background of acupuncture is open to doubt.

III

SCIENTIFIC VERSUS TRADITIONAL ACUPUNCTURE - SOME CONCLUSIONS

Acupuncture Points

In my neurophysiological theory I have explained the areas used for stimulation in acupuncture. They are partially on a roughly dermatome basis; partially involving 'long' reflexes to distant parts of the body, which implicates a distribution by specific spinal segments or nerves; and partially via unknown connections.

This theory would transform the classical small specific acupuncture point into an area as large as that of a dermatome, or to the distribution of a specific nerve, or even to an area of several dermatomes if the area has previously been hypersensitised (see chapter I). If only a few neurones are involved the skin area could be considerably smaller than a dermatome.

In most instances no doctor, even if he be an expert in acupuncture, can find an acupuncture point in those areas where there is a big expanse, such as the abdomen, back and thorax. If a group of doctors are asked to locate a specific acupuncture point in such an area, their positions will quite often vary by a considerable amount, and yet all these doctors are able to help or cure a large proportion of their patients provided they have a disease amenable to acupuncture. This suggests to me that small specific acupuncture points rarely exist, and that those researchers who have found specific types of specialised nerve endings or other structures at acupuncture points are mistaken. The structures found by these histological investigations may well be there, but they do not correspond to acupuncture points, for they do not exist. Stimulation of any layer can be effective, whether it be skin, subcutaneous tissue, muscle or periosteum. Hence one should not speak of a dermatome, but rather of a dermo-myo-sclerotome. This poses some problems, for the different layers do not always have the same segmental innervation.

In a disease of the viscera or other parts of the body there is often a reflex tenderness in the associated part of the surface. This tenderness may include muscle spasm or circulatory changes. It also presumably affects most histological structures throughout the entire depth of the appropriate area, due to their similar innervation.

As far as I know there are no specific histological elements in McBurney's point, which becomes tender in appendicitis. I think nearly every single part of the body can become reflexly tender, in a way similar to that of McBurney's point. Hence the number of acupuncture points would become infinite—indeed some books mention so many acupuncture points, that one wonders if there is any normal skin left.

McBurney's point is not a small discrete 'point', but quite a large area, whose position is somewhat variable. McBurney's point lies in the appropriate dermatome. The remainder of the dermatome is not tender or only mildly so, for as Kellgren (Fig. 9) and others have shown, certain areas within a dermatome show greater changes than others.

Some acupuncture points seem to have a constant position and may be tender even in a completely healthy person:—

G21 is situated where the trapezius arches over the first rib and hence is presumably under greater tension than other parts of the muscle.

Sp9 is located below the medial condyle, over the lower part of the medial ligament of the knee, where many women have a tender oedematous area. As this occurs nearly only in women, apart from those who have injured their knee, it is presumably hormonal. In some women this area becomes an oedematous pad of fat the size of a hand.

G20 is next to the greater occipital nerve where it arches over the occiput, just as B2 is adjacent to the supratrochlear nerve where it passes over the supraorbital ridge.

All the above and a certain number of other acupuncture points are nearly always tender, even in the healthy subject. This is probably often due to compressing a nerve trunk against the bone. Other places may be tender due to muscular tension sensitising the area and thus requiring a smaller stimulus from the acupuncture needle to be effective.

H7 is a more effective point than H3, as stimulation of H7 involves the needle piercing thicker skin and a hard ligament. This causes greater pain than needling the fatty tissue around H3 and thus obviously has stimulated more nerve fibres. For a similar reason acupuncture points which involve stimulation of the periosteum have usually a greater effect than those involving only subcutaneous fat, unless the needle is strongly twisted in the skin.

Stimulating a nerve trunk, which produces a lightning pain, is by no means more effective. In patients who have the so called cervical disc syndrome and allied conditions, stimulation of the transverse process of the 6th cervical vertebra is more effective than trying to needle the adjacent nerves of the brachial plexus.

In my experience, contrary to classical theory, the type of stimulus used in acupuncture is of little importance whether it be a needle, a thorn, an electric current, heat, a vibrator or injections. This would agree with the 'all or nothing' response of nerve fibres, which either respond or do not respond to stimulation, there being no qualitative difference. The stronger the stimulus, the greater is the effect due to activation of a larger number of neurones or their repetitive stimulation. The traditional theory that there is a qualitative difference between a hot or a cold needle, or the manner in which it is twisted or inserted, does not concur with my experience and would be harder to explain neurologically. Sometimes if the periosteum is stimulated in the region of a joint the effect is greater than if the overlying skin is needled. Possibly this is due to activation of a local reflex.

Some researchers claim there is a reduced electrical skin resistance at small discrete places, they call acupuncture points. For several years I have diligently tried to confirm this observation both in patients and cadavers. I found there are thousands of smaller or larger skin areas of reduced resistance, some of which might correspond to acupuncture, whilst most did not.

A doctor who knows acupuncture, will be able to find acupuncture points electrically, by passing the searching electrode a few times over the desired acupuncture point. Each time an active electrode is passed over the skin, it is depolarised and its electrical resistance is reduced, and if this is repeated a few times one creates, de novo, one's own electrical acupuncture point.

According to my neurophysiological theory one would not expect to find discrete acupuncture points by electrical or other means. It is possible though that larger areas, related to the distribution of groups of neurones, may be found, whilst in an abnormal state.

Meridians

In some places the course of meridians follows the pathways of nerves or the position of dermatomes, in others it does not. I have shown in chapter 1 that in most (but by no means all) instances a neurological explanation fits in with more of the observed facts than with the hypothetical meridians.

Sometimes a needle in the leg produces a sensation (not a lightning pain) along the stomach meridian where it goes over the abdomen and thorax. This does not fit in with the route taken by a nerve trunk. The connections within the spinal cord are so numerous, that further research might elucidate this and similar problems.

The experiments in chapter 1 have shown that most of the reflexes involved in acupuncture are spinal. It is possible though that some reflexes, especially those which are not instantaneous, might involve higher centres. The experiments of Downman and Koblank illustrate that more than one neural path is excited by a single stimulus. Quite possibly a single pin prick in the leg may invoke two or three separate intraspinal pathways, and also a path along the sympathetic chain. Both the intraspinal and sympathetic routes having quick responses on the target area via a spinal reflex and possibly delayed responses via suprasegmental pathways, which secondarily cause the release of hormones or vascular and other phenomena. I maintain however that the primary transmission system used in acupuncture is neural.

The fifty-nine or more meridians* described by the Chinese seem to link interdependent areas of the body, even though they may be at a considerable distance from one another. For example: A mildly stiff neck may be helped by placing a needle in a gall bladder acu-

---

* see The Meridians of Acupuncture.

puncture point on the foot, because the gall bladder meridian goes through the neck. The nervous pathway between the foot and the neck is not obvious. The ancient Chinese however linked them together by a meridian for they found the connection by experience.

The practical conclusion to be drawn from this is, that although the meridians do not exist as such, they illustrate in an almost abstract manner, the presumed neural pathways, which are as yet unknown. In that way the meridians are of paramount importance to the clinician whose main concern is to get his patients better. The meridians of acupuncture might even be compared to the meridians of geography: imaginary but useful. I hope that the investigations of neurophysiologists and others will map out the true neural pathways involved, which would then only partially correspond to meridians.

Categories of Acupuncture Points

Elsewhere it is shown that tonification and sedation, although they form a major part of traditional theory, are a philosophical conception which does not apply to the actual practice of acupuncture. If on pulse diagnosis the liver pulse is wide and hard, it is called over-active and requires sedation. If the point of sedation or tonification or any other point whatsoever on that meridian or related points on other meridians, is stimulated, the pulse on Chinese pulse diagnosis becomes normal or nearly normal. Likewise if the pulse of the liver is narrow and soft, one could call it underactive, requiring tonification. The result would be exactly the same if any of the before-mentioned points were used.

The obvious conclusion is that the twenty or so categories of acupuncture points (some books describe more categories) are superfluous. There is no physiological connection between the metal point on the heart meridian and the metal point on the liver meridian.

The different acupuncture points on the same meridian exert partly similar effects. Hence the tradition of joining them together with a line called a meridian. They have also partly dissimilar effects, for to some extent different neurons are stimulated.

Laws of Acupuncture

The various laws of acupuncture mentioned in my traditional books fall in many instances into disarray once one has discovered that tonification and sedation do not take place. Yin and Yang, coupled organs, full and empty diseases, cold and hot diseases become untenable.

The law of the five elements demonstrates some connections between organs well known to physiology, and some connections which presumably exist, but are not yet known. In clinical practice one finds that certain of the connections happen frequently, whilst the others occur rarely or never. The frequently occurring connections can in most instances be more easily explained in Western terms than via the Chinese pentagram.

If all the laws of acupuncture are taken together it will be seen that every phenomenon occurring in health and disease can be explained and hence it leaves one with little explanation at all.

A traditional Chinese doctor practising acupuncture will achieve good results, albeit for the wrong reasons, which is though of little concern to the patient: A traditional doctor may say that a specific very small acupuncture point should be stimulated; a Western doctor may say that anywhere within a given area is sufficient. Both doctors achieve equal results if the Oriental's acupuncture point lies within the area of hypersensitivity of the Westerner. Again: A Chinese doctor may say that the fire point on the Yin wood meridian should be used; his Occidental counterpart may suggest that any 'point' on the liver meridian below the knee is sufficient. The two colleagues will have equal results, for the fire point is within the Western grouping.

In certain ways the Chinese scholar, as scholars elsewhere, has made acupuncture more complicated than it really is. To this was added ancient tradition, so that the resultant medical system became a paradise of the inscrutable.

The Energy of Life—QI

The Chinese theories related to Qi (the energy of life), Nourishing Qi, Protecting Qi, Blood, Life Essence, Spirit, Fluid and similar connections mentioned in *Acupuncture: The Ancient Chinese Art of Healing*, are most easily understood as a traditional Chinese concept, linked with a view of the world different to that of most Occidentals. Western doctors who practise acupuncture, or neurophysiologists who investigate its mode of action, can do without this traditional idea.

If a patient, even a Western doctor, has been ill and then recovers, he will say 'I feel better, I have more energy'. If this same doctor is then asked what is energy (called in Chinese Qi), he will probably say that such a thing does not exist. A contradiction and at the same time not a contradiction.

From the point of view of Western medicine, disease ensues when the biochemical processes of the body are disturbed. If for example there is a deficiency of potassium, the body chemistry is altered and the patient has amongst other symptoms little energy. The energy cannot be measured directly, only its secondary effect in reducing muscular activity may be measured.

The Oriental doctor considers energy as something primary and 'real', whose deficiency causes secondarily disease. The Occidental doctor thinks the chemistry of the body is primary which only secondarily affects energy. Textbooks of physiology do not mention the conception of a biological energy as something primary.

These two points of view are only partially contradictory. They are only looking at life from a different point of view.

Much of Chinese medical theory describes what the patient feels. The patient feels differences in energy. He often feels something along the course of meridians. The Western doctor often excludes the patient's feelings and measures the serum electrolytes, haemoglobin and faecal fat instead.

Few people would disagree that when they see a meadow it is green. A physicist would say though that the meadow emits a certain wavelength of light which is then *subjectively* interpreted by the eye and brain as the colour green. This is little different from the person who is hit with a sledge hammer and then subjectively interprets it as the taste of onions—something which a Pavlov type dog could probably be trained to do.

If the physicist is asked, what a wavelength of light is, he might explain it in more detail using Einstein's particle theory of photons, which anyway is not considered to be a physical reality. From which it emerges that Chinese metaphysics is hardly less real or unreal than the theoretical background of modern physics, which is the foundation of most modern medicine.

IV

STRONG REACTORS

Certain patients respond better to acupuncture than do others. In some instances these patients are cured or their symptoms are considerably ameliorated within seconds or minutes of treatment. Both the patient and the doctor have witnessed a phenomenon which seems nearly a miracle. This chapter will describe these patients whom I have called *strong reactors* since 1962, a description which in some aspects is exaggerated in an attempt to clarify the conception.

If one looks at a strong reactor with the eye of an artist one has the impression they are *physiologically alive*; one feels as if their individual components can be moved, can be recreated—they are not an immobile statue. They are like a day in Spring, when the plants grow, the flowers blossom, the birds sing and the insects fly —not a winters day when all is static.

These patients often respond quickly or in a strong manner to the normal drugs used in orthodox medicine. They often need half, a quarter or even a tenth of the usual dose of a medicine. And if they take this small dose it works perfectly, as in the average normal patient.

On occasions I have seen a patient with hypertension, as the drug their doctor had prescribed made them feel 'like death'. Since acupuncture is rarely of benefit in hypertension, there is little benefit in trying it. If I noticed the patient was a strong reactor I would then suggest that they take a fraction of the same medicine as their general practitioner had previously prescribed for them; a dose so small that

I did not dare write it on the prescription for fear of the pharmacist's ridicule. Not infrequently this treatment worked.

Some patients who dislike orthodox medicine do so as they are the type of strong reactor for whom the average dose of a drug is an overdose. This does not apply to all drugs for they may react normally to some drugs yet strongly to others. Even the average patient reacts strongly to an occasional drug or may exhibit a rare allergy, but in the strong reactor this is more frequent. Anaesthetists who use quickly acting and powerful drugs are more aware of this problem than perhaps the average doctor.

The strong reactor responds more often than the average patient to treatment within seconds or minutes of the needle being in place. If they had symptoms these will largely or completely disappear—the headache, the painful knee, the aching back. If they came on a day they had no symptoms they may instead, if they were tense, have a feeling of a pleasant, drowsy relaxation, so that they may nearly fall asleep in the consulting room. Normally the technique which I use for stimulation in acupuncture involves twisting the needle to and fro for a minute or two causing the patient a degree of pain not dissimilar to that caused by a dentist. Despite this pain some strong reactors become soporific whilst the needle twisting is in progress. Some strong reactors may at the same time as feeling relaxed, feel more energetic, a sense akin to that of tasting the first few drops of champagne. This is different to the usual effect, of a tranquilizer for the patient is at one and the same time more relaxed and yet with an enhanced energy. Normal patients may have this relaxed feeling—with or without the champagne effect, immediately after the treatment or after a delay of a few hours; but it is not as frequent as in strong reactors.

If a needle is stuck into the foot of an average patient and twisted to and fro he may feel pain for an inch or two around the needle, unless of course a nerve trunk has been stimulated. The strong reactor on the other hand not infrequently may feel a pain going up the leg which may continue over the trunk and head on the same or opposite side. Sometimes a sensation is felt in a part of the body distant from the stimulating needle whilst the intervening section of the body is unaffected. This sensation which travels along certain paths of the body is not like the shooting electric pain felt on stimulating a major nerve trunk. It is usually fairly pleasant—as if something has just happened there. If a distant area of the body alone is affected, there is often a feeling of pleasant warmth, muscle relaxation, if the sinuses a sense of freeing and crackling. The travelling sensation is often confined to fairly narrow paths which may be centrifugal or centripetal. The sensation may travel from one end of the body to the other in one second or may take several seconds to traverse the leg. Sometimes it fits in with the course of peripheral nerves, sometimes with that of meridians (which often differs from the former), but often with neither.

Anaesthetists, acupuncturists and others who have tried to stimulate peripheral nerve trunks with a needle will know how difficult this can be, necessitating not infrequently several attempts till one is rewarded with a lightning-like pain or a muscle twitch. Surprisingly enough this is considerably easier in strong reactors, sometimes the first judicious attempt is successful. I cannot imagine the nerve trunks of strong reactors have a larger diameter. One must rather suppose that they are in a more reactive state and are more easily triggered.

Strong reactors are on the whole more sensitive people, though there are many exceptions as one may be a strong reactor from certain points of view whilst a slow reactor in other aspects. I remember seeing a colonel who had injured his neck in the Second World War. He was parachuted over Africa and spellbound as he slowly floated down to earth, by the beauty of the clouds, the forests beneath him, the intermingling of colour between light and shade. Then with a bang he suddenly hit the ground and injured his neck. Only a strong reactor would be taken in by the beauty of nature to such an extent that he forgot his own safety—the distance to the ground. Slow reactors may also be overcome by emotion, but not infrequently these emotions belong to the more basic varieties such as sex, money, hatred—though this requires very careful and often contradictory interpretation.

Strong reactors may feel it if someone is looking at them from behind, just as they may sense the atmosphere of a room when they enter it. Strong reactors are often more instinctive than the average person, for they can observe and are influenced by subtle factors to which the normal person is impervious. Many successful business people, or indeed those in many walks of life, are strong reactors. They are able to take a decision, indeed the correct decision, when only a few facts concerning the case is known to them. The ordinary person who plods along has to know all the hundred-and-one facts of a business deal before his computer-like mind, which can only digest proven facts, can function. After this long lapse of time, all other members of the business community have of course ascertained the same facts, and the business initiative of an entirely new and exclusive deal will have been lost. It will readily be apparent that some members of the academic professions are slow reactors, always requiring proof. In certain walks of life it is an advantage, even necessary, to be a slow reactor. Dr Jean Schoch of Strasbourg once said when discussing the contradiction of people's temperaments: "a symphony does not consist of equal notes".

If a patient is in favour and believes in acupuncture, it will of course tip the scales towards the strong reactor. As is readily apparent from the chapter 10* on the interplay of the mind and the body, acupuncture which acts primarily on diseases involving an easily reversible physiological process, cannot be but influenced by the mind. This does not mean that being a strong reactor is a mental process, it merely means that it is influenced by the mind.

There is a tendency for strong reactors to be neurotic, though actually only a few are. The slow reactors not infrequently are the very opposite of neurotic—possibly pedestrian machines.

Strong reactors are influenced more easily by the weather and geological conditions. Those who feel heavenly in Aberdeen and lethargic in London (or vice versa) are more likely to be strong reactors. Likewise those who respond strongly to the special winds one has in some countries such as the Föhn in the southern Alps.

There is no definite division between the strong and slow reactor. The proportion of each in the general population depends entirely on the criteria one uses. From a purely practical and clinical point of view one could say that about 5% of the population are hyper-strong reactors. Hyper-strong reactors and strong reactors counted together might form 10% or even 30% of the population if one is generous.

Acupuncture anaesthesia (really analgesia) works only, in my experience (though others who are experts disagree) in the hyper-strong reactor. In 1974 I reported the results of a hundred experiments in acupuncture analgesia and come to the conclusion that it

* of Acupuncture: The Ancient Chinese Art of Healing.

worked reasonably though not perfectly, in 10% of patients. Since then I have come to the conclusion that the criteria I used were a little optimistic and the figure should be revised to a mere 5%. Some experiments* were performed which showed that the acupuncture analgesia was an objective and not a psychosomatic phenomenon, in the few in whom it worked.

On a few occasions I have had the impression that people who have changed from a mixed diet to that of a vegetarian, have started to react more strongly. This of course often goes hand in hand with an altered outlook on life, which includes being more receptive to the finer things of life, and hence this latter reason might be more important than the change in diet.

Despite many years of experience and interest, I still find that I am only right in some three out of four instances when deciding who is a strong reactor—as measured subsequently by the strength of response to treatment.

In the practice of acupuncture I find it quite important to know who is, and who is not a strong reactor. The strong reactor needs a gentle treatment in acupuncture, just as he needs a small dose of medicine when looked after by orthodox means. In the extreme case it may be sufficient to prick in only one place, with a fine needle to a depth of one millimetre, for one second. In the average strong reactor one or two pairs of needles are sufficient, and they should be twisted with about a quarter of the severity normally employed. If one wishes to stimulate a larger number of places this should be done even more gently. One might compare the dose of acupuncture given to the average adult strong reactor, as the same as one might give to a five-year-old child who is a normal reactor. In this connection it should be added that the easiest way to measure the dose of acupuncture is to compare it to the total pain caused to the patient.

If a strong reactor is treated too vigorously either the treatment does not work, or he has a reaction (see Chapter 10†), which usually consists of a temporary worsening of the patient's symptoms. This is unpleasant but passes off in minutes, hours or days, according to the case. In say migraine a reaction is unpleasant but of no import-

* Mann, Felix. Acupuncture Analgesia, report of 100 experiments. British Journal of Anaesthia, 1974, 46: 361–4.

† of Acupuncture: The Ancient Chinese Art of Healing.

ance. In asthma and some other diseases, it would be of importance and hence such patients should at the first consultation be treated very gently and with caution, in case they are strong reactors.

Those doctors who are particularly interested in such matters, might observe that in some hyper-strong reactors the doctor may have a mild prickly sensation over the whole of his body in the presence of a hyper-strong reactor. At least this is my experience.

Women, who as a rule have more intuition than men, are likewise more often strong reactors. Before a man will do something he has to understand it; whilst a woman will act on a hunch—and be more often right. In the days when I worked as a junior doctor in a hospital I remember how often the intellectual doctor who judged his patient on laboratory results, was not infrequently eclipsed by the Ward Sister who had little technical knowledge but a heart that judged a patient by his smile.

In deciding if a patient is likely to be a strong reactor or not one has to take many contradictory facets into account, for people are made of contradictions. Whatever is decided can only be tentative till one actually sees the result of treatment. It is therefore sometimes advisable to try an initial tentative gentle treatment.

V

SEGMENTAL AND GENERAL
SYMPATHETIC RESPONSE

Sato and Schmidt* have shown that stimulation of a peripheral nerve, as is done in the everyday practice of acupuncture, has two results. There is a quick effect on the sympathetics of the same and neighbouring segments, and a delayed general sympathetic stimulation of the whole body which originates supraspinally from the sympathetic reflex centres.

Seven cats were anaesthetized and the following nerves or dorsal roots were dissected and mounted for stimulation on electrodes: the intercostals T3 and T4, the spinal nerves L1 to L4, the dorsal roots of L7 and S1, and various nerves inervating the skin and muscles of the hind leg. Recording electrodes were placed on the white ramus communicans of T3, T4 and L1, L2 (Fig. 18).

In the experiments the above mentioned intercostal nerves, spinal nerves, dorsal roots or leg peripheral nerves were stimulated differently according to the experiment, ranging from threshold level to fifty times threshold. The recording electrode or the white ramus communicans measured the preganglionic sympathetic outflow in that particular segment.

At threshold stimulation x 50, the following recordings (Fig. 19) were made, representing in each case for clarity the average computerised record of several experiments. The recording was done only from the L1 white ramus communicans.

* Sato, A., and Schmidt, R. F. Spinal and supraspinal components of the reflex discharges into lumbar and thoracic white rami. Journal of Physiology, 1971, 212: 839–850. Also drawings in this chapter.

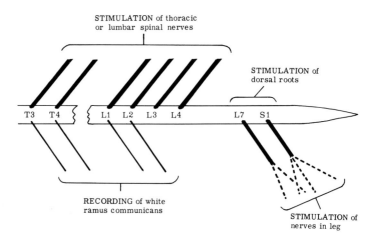

STIMULATION of thoracic
or lumbar spinal nerves

STIMULATION of
dorsal roots

T3   T4   L1   L2   L3   L4   L7   S1

RECORDING of white
ramus communicans

STIMULATION of
nerves in leg

Fig. 18

WHITE RAMI REFLEXES

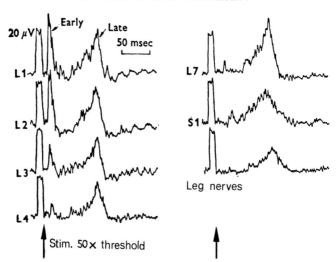

20 µV   Early   Late
50 msec

L1

L2

L3

L4

Stim. 50 × threshold

L7

S1

Leg nerves

Fig. 19

It will be noticed that in most records the sympathetic reflex discharges fall into two groups: an early and a late, separated by some 50 milliseconds.

The early discharge becomes smaller the further the stimulus is removed from that of the recording segment L1. In contrast, the late component had a rather constant size whether spinal nerves, dorsal roots or cutaneous nerves of the hind limb (the sacral nerve) were stimulated.

The latency of the early discharge increased the further the stimulated segment was from L1. The latency of the late discharge increased only fractionally as the distance to the medullary sympathetic centres was only slightly increased.

The late discharge, which represents the general sympathetic response of the body, is elicited at lower levels of stimulation, for it is activated with a stimulus of 1.5 of the threshold value, whilst the early discharge requires 5, though this can vary according to the state of the animal.

When a recording was made from either the thoracic or lumbar white rami communicans, and then the cervical cord was divided or infiltrated with local anaesthetic at C1, the late discharge disappeared. Thus it is apparent that this is a supraspinal component.

Response in Specific Areas and not in others

If the pulmonary vein-atrial junction in a dog is stimulated there is* :

1. Increased activity in the cardiac sympathetics
2. Decreased activity in the renal sympathetics
3. No alteration in the activity of the abdominal sympathetics below the level of the renal artery.

The above suggests that although there may be a local segmental sympathetic response in addition to a generalised delayed sympathetic response, as described by Sato and Schmidt; there are in addition specific areas that may respond in a positive or negative manner or even remain neutral.

* Karin, F., Kidd, C., Malpas, C. M., Penna, P. E. The Effects of stimulation of the left atrial receptors on sympathetic efferent nerve fibres. Proceedings of the Journal of Physiology, 1971, 213: 38P–39P.

VI

DERMATOMES, MYOTOMES, SCLEROTOMES

Reference of Pain and Tenderness when muscle is Stimulated

J. H. Kellgren has made many experiments* which are confirmed by the everyday practice of acupuncture. As a stimulus he injected 0.1 to 0.3 cc of 6% sodium chloride intramuscularly, which produces a severe pain lasting several minutes. In acupuncture the stimulus is usually less severe, or if severe is due to stimulation of the skin, so that the reference of pain mentioned in the ensuing paragraphs is not so often noticed.

If the gluteus medius in the upper part of the buttock is stimulated, a diffuse pain is felt over the lower part of the buttock and back of the thigh (Fig. 20).

If the upper part of the tibialis anterior is stimulated, there is often a diffuse pain in the whole of the belly of the muscle and also over the instep (Fig. 21).

Kellgren also injected saline into the multifidus opposite the 9th thoracic spine, into the intercostal muscles of the 9th intercostal space in the mid axillary line, and into the rectus abdominus 3 cm above the umbilicus. The pain from all three was referred to roughly the same area near the mid dorsal line and the mid central line (Fig. 22). Interestingly though, the pain from the multifidus was felt

* Kellgren, J. H. Observations on referred pain arising from muscle. Clinical Science, 1938–9, 3 : 175–190. Also drawings in this chapter.

Ibid. On the distribution of pain arising from deep somatic structures with charts of segmental pain areas. Clinical Science 1939–42, 4 : 35–46.

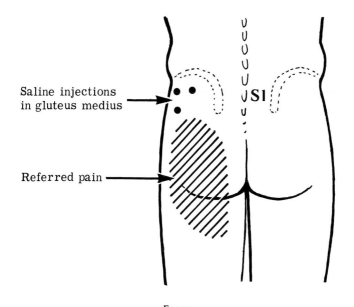

Saline injections in gluteus medius

Referred pain

FIG. 20

mainly in the back and less ventrally, that from the rectus abdominus mainly ventrally and to a lesser extent posteriorly, whilst the mid axillary line intercostal injection was felt equally in front and at the back.

If the testis is firmly compressed between fingers and thumb, the pain is first felt in the scrotum, the pain radiating to the groin and lower lumbar region only on increased pressure. If saline is injected into the multifidus opposite the space between the 1st and 2nd lumbar spines, there is severe pain in the back which radiates to a lesser extent to the groin and scrotum. When the internal obliques are stimulated near the anterior superior iliac spine, the pain is felt mainly in this region, but is also referred as a slight pain to the lower lumbar area and the testes (Fig. 23).

In most of Kellgren's experiments, the reference of pain remained within the same myotome. If the stimulation was extremely strong the referred pain might spread one segment above and below. When

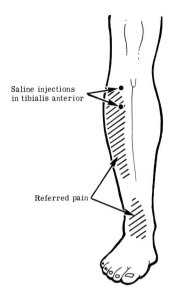

Fɪɢ. 21

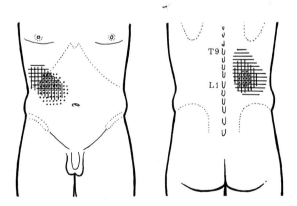

Fɪɢ. 22 Multifidus horizontal hatching, intercostals vertical hatching, rectus abdominis stippling

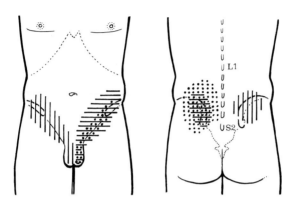

FIG. 23 Testis vertical hatching, abdominal obliques horizontal hatching, multifidus stippling.

long muscles, which span several segments, such as the sacro-spinials or rectus abdominus were stimulated, the pain often spread to several segments.

According to Kellgren the areas of referred pain near the mid ventral and mid dorsal lines, correspond to the area where the anterior and posterior primary divisions of the spinal nerves emerge from the skeletal musculature.

Kellgren differentiated the superficial and deep muscular pain as follows: he injected a muscle belly and obtained distant referred superficial pain and deep tenderness in the same region. If local anaesthetic was injected intradermally, both persisted; when injected deeply, the tenderness on pressure disappeared, whilst the superficial pain remained.

Kellgren came to the conclusion that there are three main layers of the body concerned with pain distribution:

1. When the skin is stimulated, there is normally very accurate localisation of the pain, which is also confined to a small area—unless the stimulus is unusually strong.

2. The middle layer consists of the more superficially placed deep structures: the deep fascia enclosing the limbs and trunk; and any periosteum, ligament or tendon sheath which is situated sub-cutaneously. This layer when stimulated causes pain over a somewhat

larger area, an area which may encompass the site of stimulation or
even lie at a small distance from it.

3. Apart from the above there are all the deeper layers which if
stimulated give rise to diffuse pain of more or less segmental distribution. This pain is more markedly segmental when arising from the
interspinus ligaments, intercostal spaces and deep structures of the
trunk and limb girdles. The pain is more local from the extremities
and joints. There is a tendency for pain which arises in a limb muscle,
to be referred to the joint which the muscle moves, provided it is in
the same segment.

The importance to acupuncture of Kellgren's research will be
apparent from other sections of the book. If it is possible, when
treating a patient to elicit a referred pain, the result is usually better.
If in addition it is possible from a distant pin prick, to cause a
referred pain in the area of the patients' symptoms or pathology,
the result will be even still better.

Many authors such as Janet Travell have written on this subject
indeed every doctor who practises acupuncture using a deep needling
technique must notice it every day of his practice. It is such a
common observation that few I think would deny it.

Comparison of Areas of Reference

The foregoing pages demonstrate the importance to acupuncture of
areas of reference, those differing according to the tissue stimulated
—dermatome, myotome, sclerotome, vasculartome. The method of
investigation is also important: hyposensitivity from loss of function
of a single nerve root, electrical skin resistance in sympathectomcised
patients, electrical skin resistance on stimulation of anterior spinal
roots, pain distribution after hypertomic saline injection of interspinous ligaments. There is also the distribution of the peripheral
nerves and also of the sympathetics, though the later probably
largely corresponds to the vasculartome.

Once all these areas of reference are taken into account, most of
which can be understood from a Western medical point of view, I
am sure meridians will be relegated to history.

Many of the books or articles describing reference areas are not
too easily accessible to everyone, and hence l am reproducing them
here to facilitate use.

The Dermatomes from Keegan and Garrett

Figs. 24, 25 and 26 from: Keegan, J. J. and Garrett, F. D. The segmental distribution of the cutaneous nerves in the limbs of man. *Anatomical Record*, 1948, 102: 409-439.

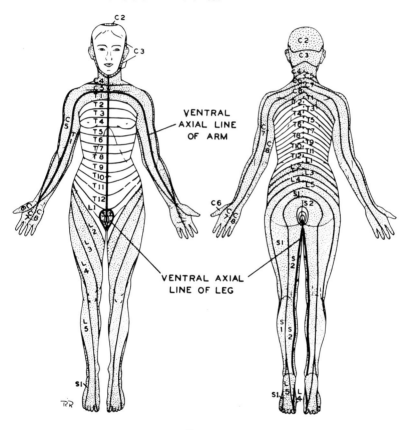

VENTRAL
AXIAL LINE
OF ARM

VENTRAL AXIAL
LINE OF LEG

FIG. 24

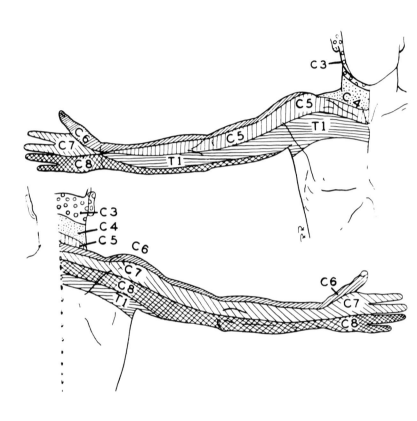

FIG. 25

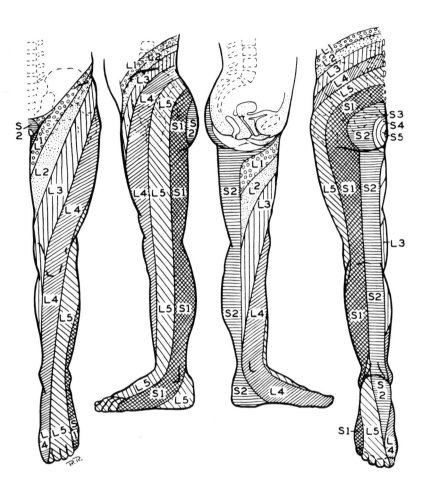

FIG. 26

Deep Pain Reference from Thomas Lewis

Fig. 27. Lewis, T. The segmental areas of deep pain developed by the injection of the corresponding interspinous ligament, with hypertonic saline. *Pain*, 1942, The Macmillan Co., New York.

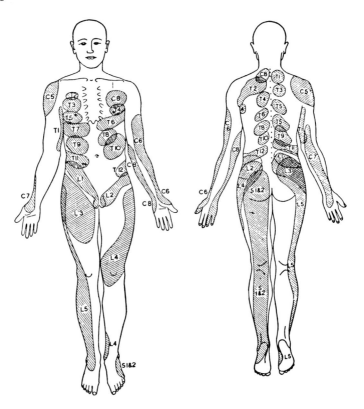

FIG. 27

Dermatomes, Myotomes and Sclerotomes from Inman and Saunders

Figs. 28, 29, 30 and 31. Inmann, V. T. and Saunders, J. B. de C. Referred pain from skeletal structures. *Journal of Nervous Mental Diseases*, 1944, 99: 660-667. Copyright 1944, The Williams and Wilkins Co., Baltimore. Slightly modified by Chusid, J. G.

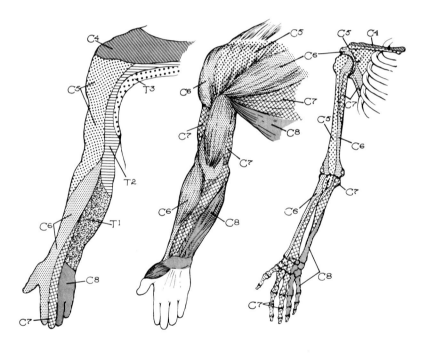

FIG. 28

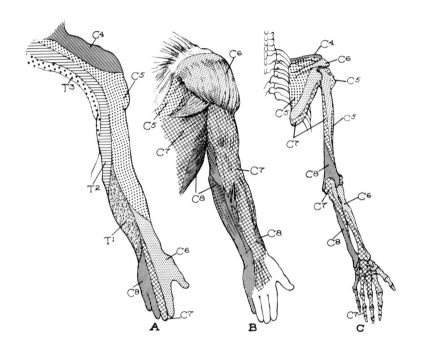

Fig. 29

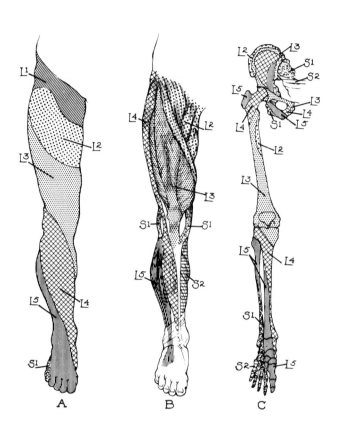

FIG. 30

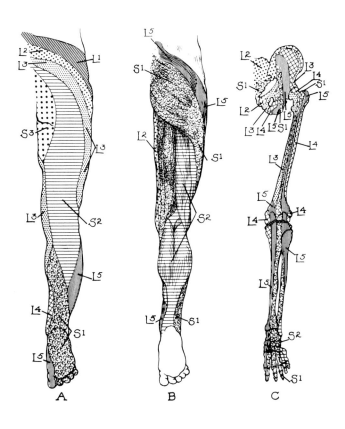

FIG. 31

Trigger Areas and Pain Reference Patterns from Janet Travell

Figs. 32, 33, 34, 35 and 36. Travell, J. Temperomandibular joint pain referred from muscles of the head and neck. *Journal of Prosthetic Dentistry*, 1960, Vol. 10, No. 4: 745-763.

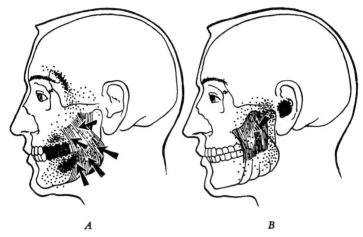

A   B

FIG. 32 Pain reference patterns of the masseter muscle: *A*, Superficial layer. *B*, Deep layer. Trigger areas are indicated by arrows, and their pain reference zones by the stippled and black regions

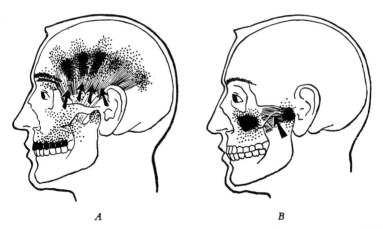

A   B

FIG. 33 *A*. Composite pain reference pattern of the temporalis muscle. Trigger areas are indicated by arrows, and their reference zones by the stippled and black regions. *B*, Composite pain reference pattern of the external pterygoid muscle

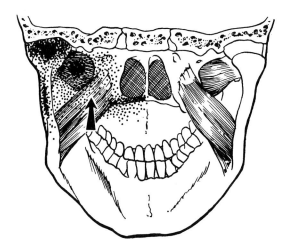

FIG. 34 Composite pain reference pattern of the internal pterygoid muscle. A partial coronal section is shown with a view of the external and internal pterygoid muscles from the back of the mouth. Trigger areas at the arrow in the internal pterygoid muscle refer pain to the stippled regions. (Based on drawing by Netter, F.: Anatomy of the Mouth, Clin. Symp. 10: 76, 1958.)

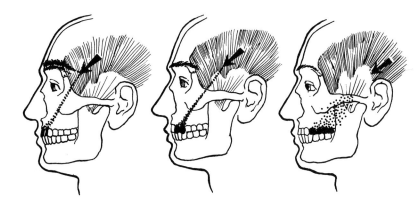

FIG. 35 Specific trigger areas at three sites in the temporalis muscle, as observed in a case of facial neuralgia. Trigger areas were located at arrows, and pain was referred to the black and stippled zones

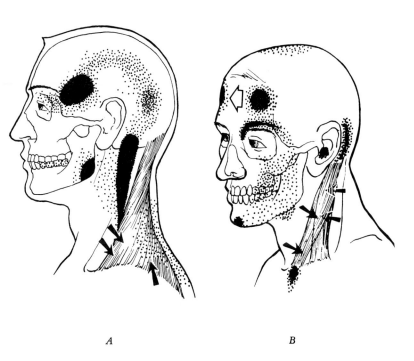

A   B

Fig. 36 *A*, Composite pain reference pattern of the trapezius muscle, suprascapular region. Trigger areas are indicated by arrows, and pain reference zones by the stippled and black regions.

B, Composite pain reference patterns of the clavicular and sternal divisions of the sterno-mastoid. The sternal division refers pain mainly to the cheek, eyebrow, pharynx, tongue, chin, throat, and sternum. The clavicular division refers pain mainly to the forehead bilaterally, to the posterior auricular region and deep in the ear, and infrequently to the teeth. Trigger areas are indicated by arrows, and pain reference zones by the stippled and black regions.

Fig. 37. Travell, J. Factors affecting pain of injection. *Journal of the American Medical Association*, 1955, 158: 368-371. Copyright 1955, American Medical Association.

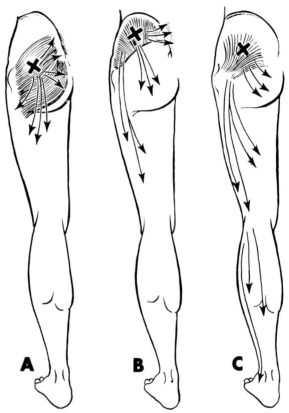

FIG. 37 Distribution of referred pain evoked by needle when inserted into trigger areas (*X*) located at common sites of intramuscular injections. Referred pain is most intense in region of arrowheads. *A*, gluteus maximus muscle. *B*, gluteus medius muscle. *C*, gluteus minimus muscle after removal of gluteus maximus and medius muscles

Fig. 38. Travell, J. Referred pain from skeletal muscle. *New York State Journal of Medicine*, 1955, 55: 331339. Fig. 38 and captions reprinted by permission from the *New York State Journal of Medicine*, copyright by the Medical Society of the State of New York.

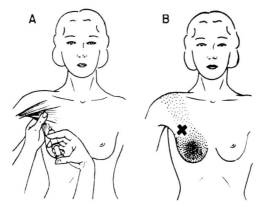

FIG. 38 Breast syndrome of pectoralis major muscle; *A*, manner of holding muscle for local procaine infiltration; *B*, distribution of pain (stippled) from trigger area (X), induced either by compressing it between the fingers or by inserting needle as shown in *A*

Trigger Points and Pain Distribution from Anders Sola

Figs. 39, 40, 41, 42 and 43. Sola, A. E. and Williams, R. L. Myofasicial pain syndromes. *Neurology*, 1956, Vol. 6, No. 2: 91-95. Reprinted from *Neurology*, © 1956 by Harcourt Brace Jovanovich, Inc.

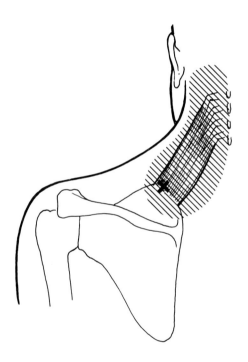

FIG. 39 The attachments of the levator scapulae muscle are shown and the common location of the trigger point is indicated by the cross. The hatched area represents the common distribution of pain in this syndrome

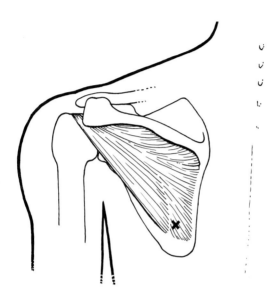

FIG. 40 The attachments of the infraspinatus muscle are shown and the common location of the trigger point is indicated by the cross

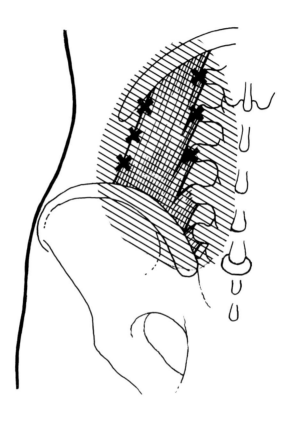

FIG. 41 The attachments and landmarks around the quadratus lumborum are shown. The crosses indicate common locations of trigger points in this syndrome. The hatched area represents the usual area of pain

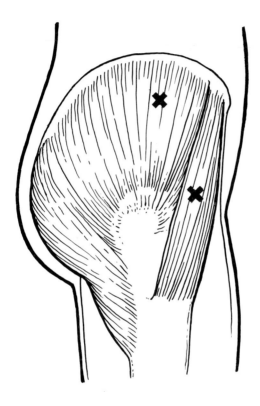

FIG. 42 The attachments of the tensor fascia lata and the gluteus medius are shown. The crosses indicate the common locations of trigger points

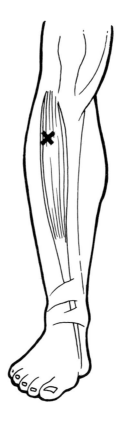

FIG. 43 The attachments of the anterior tibialis and the common location of the trigger point
are shown

Dermatomes of Referred Pain from Lumbosacral and Pelvic Joint Ligaments from George Hackett

Fig. 44. Hackett, G. S. Joint ligament relaxation treated by fibro-osseous proliferation, 1956. Charles C. Thomas, Springfield, Illinois. From Homans, John. A textbook of surgery, 6th Ed., 1945. Courtesy of Charles C. Thomas, Springfield, Illinois.

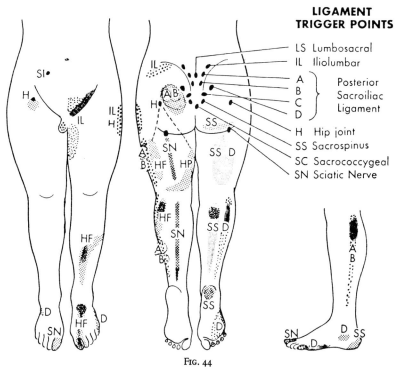

LIGAMENT TRIGGER POINTS

LS Lumbosacral
IL Iliolumbar
A }
B } Posterior
C } Sacroiliac
D } Ligament
H Hip joint
SS Sacrospinus
SC Sacrococcygeal
SN Sciatic Nerve

FIG. 44

IL Iliolumbar ligament (ilial attachment) abdomen, groin, genitalia, buttock, thigh (inner anterior)
AB Posterior sacroiliac ligament (upper 2/3rds) buttock, thigh, leg (outer surface)
D Posterior sacroiliac ligament (lower outer fibers) thigh, leg (outer calf), foot (outer margin and sole to 5-4-3-2 toes accompanied by sciatica, loss of ankle reflex and body list)
HP Hip articular ligament (posterior superior fibers, pelvic attachment) thigh (posterior medial)
HF Hip, articular ligament (posterior superior fibers, femoral attachment) thigh, upper half of leg (lateral to calf), lower half of leg (anterior to tibia), top of foot to big toe and half 2nd toe
SS Sacrospinus and sacrotuberus ligament (sacral attachment) thigh, central calf of leg, heel
SN 'Sciatica'—nerve pain accompanying relaxed ligaments (lower end of sacroiliac joint)

VII

SOME PHILOSOPHICAL CONSIDERATIONS

In Chapter XI of *Acupuncture: The Ancient Chinese Art of Healing*, it was shown that in general the diseases which are amenable to acupuncture are those which are physiologically reversible: asthma may be cured whilst emphysema is irreversible, likewise a duodenal ulcer is reversible whilst an hour glass stomach is not. Some diseases with an irreversible pathology may be indirectly alleviated: low backache and sciatica presumably respond due to the altered tone of the lumbar muscles slightly altering the position of the vertebrae and hence alleviating nerve root pressure.

It is readily apparent that many of the diseases mentioned in the above paragraph and in Chapter XI are what are nowadays called psychosomatic, and as such are unfortunately considered by many doctors as not 'real'—meaning not organic disease. The patient who has these 'unreal' diseases is often given a tranquiliser, an aspirin or a sympathetic pat on the back.

A 'real' organic disease is, since the days of Virchow, considered to be, in the majority of cases, one in which there are *changes in cellular pathology*. More recently gross changes in chemical pathology have been added. If one excludes acute disease (which is barely mentioned in this chapter) this presents a nihilistic dilemma:

'Real' diseases are only recognised as such, if there are accompanying pathological changes when, as a rule the condition is irreversible because the regenerative ability of chronically diseased tissue in man is extremely low—not as in the lower animals. In short: *once a chronic disease is diagnosed it is by definition incurable.*

Orthodox Western medicine is in the same nihilistic dilemma. A surgeon may excise the area of pathological change, but he does not cure. Insulin may alleviate the symptoms of diabetes, but the patient is not cured because the day he does not take insulin he is as ill as before. The achievements of surgery and drugs should not be underestimated, for innumerable lives are saved or disease alleviated, by their use. But, at the same time, it is clear that, in most instances, they do not cure—in the sense that changes in cellular pathology are not usually reversed.

Likewise acupuncture does not cure 'real' diseases. The temporary alleviation which is achieved by taking a medicine every day, cannot be emulated by acupuncture, for acupuncture is normally only applied half a dozen times, followed sometimes by a few single follow-up treatments.

The aim of acupuncture, and I hope that of Western medicine in the future, is to treat disease before it is by definition incurable. But since most 'real' diseases are incurable, what can one do?

I think that most chronic diseases with obvious changes in cellular pathology are preceded by a preclinical phase of perhaps many years duration. I cannot imagine that someone who has diabetes, hypertension or malignant disease one year, was really healthy the year before. In most of these diseases there was probably some mild physiological dysfunction of many years' duration, which only finally culminated in changes in cellular pathology or gross biochemistry.

It is this early stage of a mild physiological dysfunction, still presumably reversible, which doctors should try to treat. Since this preclinical phase of disease cannot be diagnosed by conventional methods, one has to think of a different approach.

A large proportion, if not the majority, of patients seen by a general practitioner have diseases which many doctors consider 'unreal', 'psychosomatic', 'functional', 'supratentorial', 'neuro-vegetative disequilibrium'. The hospital consultant sees less patients with 'unreal' diseases, as the general practitioner tries to refer only 'real' diseases to him. In the final analysis the doctor will insist that his diagnosis of a 'supratentorial' disease was correct for at autopsy a patient who has had symptoms for thirty years and died at eighty will probably show no unexpected pathological changes.

I personally think that most patients who have symptoms have a disease, whether there is any pathology there or not. I find that the proportion of hysterics who should be excluded from the above considerations is exceedingly small—and even they should be cured of their hysteria. I see no reason whatsoever why the average person should invent a disease, why they should invent that they are tired till halfway through the morning, that they do not have the energy to enjoy their work or leisure. Many perfectly normal citizens have vague symptoms such as the above for perhaps half their life. They often do not tell their doctor as they resent his depreciating reception of their psychosomatic symptoms.

Chinese pulse diagnosis* can, not infrequently, find a dysfunction in these patients with 'supratentorial' disease. With the appropriate treatment the 'supratentorial' disease is alleviated or cured and the patient's fatigue, lethargy, restlessness or other symptoms, which he may have had for many years, are dissipated. In these cases acupuncture is sometimes the appropriate treatment, in other cases less food and running a mile before breakfast is the answer.

I think, though I have no proof, that if this preclinical stage of disease is cured it prevents the later development of an obvious disease with pathology. Sometimes a disease may remain at the preclinical stage and develop no further.

In modern medicine, *pathology* is the Queen of Sciences. In the system I am proposing, the *symptoms* of the patient would achieve paramount importance. I believe the human being is more sensitive than a test tube. And a doctor should learn how to evaluate the minutest of symptoms or the slightest change in the bearing or temperament of his patient, making medicine once more an art. Later, when there are chemical and cellular changes, science takes over from that probing, intuitive art.

A not inconsiderable number of doctors, would classify amongst the 'unreal' or 'psychosomatic' diseases, migraine, ulcerative colitis, hay fever and duodenal ulcer. If a method of treatment is able to help these diseases it is often considered little more than hypnosis. Brain tumours and broken bones are the business of 'real' medicine.

The human body though, does not function along purely physical or purely mental paths; usually there will be interaction. If one has had a fright it is normal to have palpitations; those who do not are

* see Chapter IX of Acupuncture: The Ancient Chinese Art of Healing.

considered superhuman or subnormal. If someone vomits at table it is usual for the others present to lose their appetite, with diminished salivary secretion. It is quite normal for young men and women to have not only a mental effect on one another but also some physiological effect—and when this never happens, it is considered abnormal.

It is similar in disease. It is normal for the mind and body to interact. If a disease can no longer be influenced by the mind it is often very advanced with marked pathological changes, making it a 'real' disease which is incurable. In congestive cardiac failure, the cardiac muscle is probably irreparably hypertrophied. Hence this process can no longer be influenced by the mind. Digitalis will help for a day, but the congestive cardiac failure could only have been cured at the preclinical phase, at which stage both the mind, acupuncture and drugs can influence it.

Many consider that a double blind cross over trial can distinguish between a real medicine and a placebo, because the effect of the mind is excluded. This is to a large extent correct in modern medicines with their strong pharmacological actions: pentothal works or it does not work; when it is excreted the effect wears off and more has to be injected. Pentothal presumably temporarily blocks one link in the biochemical chain. Vitamin B12 temporarily replaces a deficiency. If normal medicines are to function properly they have to be more or less continuously present in the body.

The opposite holds true with the more biological and pre-clinical type of medicine I am advocating. In acupuncture one only stimulates (via the nervous system) the body a few times, so that afterwards it functions normally and does not require the continuous administration of medicines or acupuncture. As this is a *weak* physiological rather than a *strong* pharmacological effect it probably also requires the synergistic action of the mind and hence a double blind cross over trial has little meaning under these circumstances.

Alexander Macdonald* and colleagues have shown that part of the effect of acupuncture is physiological and part mental. This is of course true of everything in medicine: in surgery and when using modern powerful drugs, the physiological effect usually domin-

*Macdonald, A.J.R., Macrae, K.D., Masters, B.R. Rubin, A.P. Superficial acupuncture in the relief of chronic low back pain: a placebo controlled randomised trial. Annals of the Royal College of Surgeons of England, 1983, 65: 44–46.

Fig. 45 Mean percentage reductions

Patient groups	% pain relief after each treatment	% pain score reduction	% activity pain score reduction	% physical signs reduction	% severity and pain area reduction	Combined average % reduction
(a) Acupuncture (N = 8)	77.35	57.15	52.04	96.78	73.75	71.41
(b) Placebo (N = 9)	30.14	22.74	5.83	29.17	18.89	21.35
	**	—	*	**	**	**

Significance assessed by the Wilcoxon Rank-sum tests
*   p < 0.05
** p < 0.01
— not significant

ates; whilst in the practice of the average general practitioner, the physiological and mental effects are of probably more equal importance. *Backache*

Macdonald studied seventeen consecutive patients whose chronic low back pain failed to derive sufficient relief from appropriate conventional methods of treatment. The cases were severe enough to be referred from the orthopaedic or rheumatic departments to a pain relief clinic. They were diagnosed as having: anterior spondylitis, ankylosing spondylitis, degenerative disc lesion, non-articular rheumatism, osteoarthritis, prolapsed intervertebral disc, arachnoiditis, sacro-iliac ligamentous strain, Scheuermann's osteochondritis or ideopathic. There was random allocation of patients with regard to disease, age and sex.

In each patient five measures of treatment efficiency were recorded, subjectively or objectively and the improvement or otherwise in each case, noted by an independent observer.

One group of patients were treated by superficial acupuncture, in which the needle only pierces the skin and subcutaneous fat.

The placebo group were treated by the biggest and most impressive looking machine in the hospital, with many dials and flashing lights, whose cooling system made a whirring sound. Electrodes from this machine were applied to similar parts of the body to those which had been needled by acupuncture. The machine was regulated, though, in such a way, that when it was switched on, no current flowed through the electrodes.

The table (Fig. 45) shows that the acupuncture is some three times as effective as only placebo. Interestingly three patients were temporarily worse after placebo treatment, though this did not happen at subsequent treatments which were deliberately of shorter duration.

VIII

FAILED RESEARCH

When I first studied acupuncture in 1958, many doctors thought that one could locate acupuncture points electrically. It was said that the electrical skin resistance, or impedance, was reduced at an acupuncture point. Hence it was a relatively simple matter of a patient holding an earthed electrode in one hand, whilst the doctor ran a searching electrode over the area of skin where he thought he would find an acupuncture point. It was frequently further postulated, that if an acupuncture point were 'active', that is requiring stimulation, the electrical skin resistance was reduced by an even greater amount than with a 'non-active' acupuncture point. A few doctors, also claimed that the resistance was reduced along the course of the meridians, albeit to a lesser extent than with the active or non-active acupuncture points.

Filled with the enthusiasm of youth, and the uncritical childlike belief that many people have at some time in their lives, I bought what I thought was the best commercially available electrical acupuncture point detector: an apparatus which I bought in the belief that it would work and help to provide some scientific basis for acupuncture.

I found that however diligently I tried using this apparatus, I could detect neither acupuncture points, whether active or inactive, nor meridians. Subsequently I bought two more electrical acupuncture point detectors with the same dismal result. Over the years several dozen different models have been made by various manufacturers, some of which I have tested whilst looking at the manufacturers' displays at acupuncture conferences. But always, to my inexplicable consternation, the acupuncture point proved elusive.

It was only gradually that I realised, as I have described in this book, that acupuncture points and meridians do not exist—at least in the traditionally accepted sense. During the time when this gradual change in my conception of acupuncture was taking place, I met Professor Bernard Watson, Dr Stuart Meldrum and their colleagues many of whom were physicists, at the Department of Medical Electronics at St Bartholomew's Hospital, London. Some of the lines of research mentioned in this chapter evolved through our mutual discussions.

Electrical Skin Resistance Measurements

McCarroll and Rowley* made a grid five units in length and five in width, so that a large square enclosed 25 small squares. This 25 square grid was placed in various positions on the arm where some of the traditional acupuncture points were located. The searching electrode, which was one millimetre in diameter, incorporated a soft spring, so that the electrode, whatever its position, applied a constant force of 0.1 kgm/mm² to the skin.

Measurement of the electrical impedance in all 25 squares was made in a random manner, on several occasions, with the grid in various positions. No particular areas of reduced electrical skin impedance were found, except where the electrode impinged on a hard object—bone or tendon.

It was also found that when the electrode was applied to the same place for 20 seconds, the impedance was reduced by some 50%. Beyond this point the impedance was suddenly reduced by 94% of its original value—it was considered that the protein mat of the stratum corneum had been torn.

The above experiment confirms my own experience: If one is searching for an 'acupuncture point', the longer one looks, i.e. the longer one presses the electrode over the same area, the more likely is one to create due to the apparatus, a non-existent acupuncture

*McCarroll, G. Duncan and Rowley, Blair A. An investigation of the existance of electrically located acupuncture points. Transactions on Biomedical Engineering, 1979, 26–3: 177–181.

point. If one passes the electrode over the skin in a regular, but random manner, no obvious correlation exists between the variations in impedance and traditional acupuncture points.

The impedance is sometimes reduced over superficial veins, if an electrode without a spring is pressed harder against the skin, by perspiration, or over a boney prominence. Also some types of skin have a lower impedance. The sudden breakdown in the electrical skin resistance, referred to above, may easily be observed if an electrode is pressed a little harder than usual.

In the case of either a disease of the viscera or spasm of the skeletal muscle, one would expect reflex changes in the skin, due to the viscero-cutaneous or muscular-cutaneous reflexes, mentioned earlier in this book. One would likewise expect these reflex changes to affect various properties of the skin, possibly including the electrical resistance or impedance.

One would however, I think, expect to find quite large areas of skin exhibiting these electrical changes, such as the reflexly tender areas, often the size of a hand, mentioned by Kellgren (see Chapter I, Fig. 9). Possibly the area might even be larger affecting a substantial part of a dermatome, myotome or vasculartome. If a sympathectomy is performed, many nerves have to be divided to produce vascular dilation and a large area of reduced electrical skin impedance. If only a few nerves are divided there is not a correspondingly reduced result, but no result at all.

It is thus apparent, that the researcher should look for *large areas* of skin exhibiting electrical (or other) changes, *which are only present in disease or dysfunction*. Searching for tiny acupuncture points, which are present on both the healthy and diseased body is probably a science-fiction interpretation of certain traditional ideas, which have proved erroneous.

Infra Red Photography

It is often possible to relieve a patient's symptoms within a few seconds or minutes of treatment by acupuncture. It seemed reasonable to suppose that if a patient had headache, pain in the neck and shoulders or pain over the sinuses, and these symptoms were alleviated, that there would be evidence of an altered bloodflow in the affected region and that this could be demonstrated by infra red photography.

Ten friends, patients or members of the department with a variety of symptoms volunteered for the experiment. In some instances the acupuncture alleviated their symptoms, in others it did not. In no instance was there a significant alteration in the infra red photographs, taken before and after the experiment. Even in those patients who had instantaneous relief of symptoms, the changes in the infra red photographs were neither sufficiently significant nor were they consistent.

Other researchers, who have published their results, claim to have found significant changes on their investigation by infra red photography. This is contrary to our experience. It should be remembered though that it is quite easy to have erroneous changes. This may be due to the patient not having reached a stable temperature in a stable environment of sufficient duration. Emotional response easily changes skin temperature as can be demonstrated by bio-feedback techniques. It is also possible to achieve an occasional change, which is difficult to repeat.

Electromyography

Many patients have stiff, tender and painful shoulders. If these are successfully treated by acupuncture, and the shoulders are examined before and after treatment, the doctor may find the shoulders feel softer, giving the impression the muscles are more relaxed.

It seems that many patients suffering from low backache may have spasm of the sacrospinalis, which is relaxed after successful treatment. Such patients may be unable to touch their toes when standing with their knees straight, but are able to do so after treatment; presumably due to muscle relaxation.

It should therefore have been easy to demonstrate the effect of acupuncture by electromyography. In all these experiments the recording was done with surface electrodes over the afflicted area, so that there was little disturbance of the affected musculature or the overlying or adjacent tissue. For the same reason the acupuncture was performed in the hands or feet, as these are at some distance from the site of the symptoms: the shoulders or lumbo-sacral area.

Twelve friends and patients with the above symptoms were

needled in the appropriate place in the hands or feet, sometimes the feet were used to alleviate the symptoms in the shoulders.

Over 50% of the patients responded within a few seconds of treatment. The symptoms (and presumably the muscle spasm) remained better for a shorter or longer period in each individual. In not one instance was the electromyograph altered by acupuncture.

The electromyograph used was the EMG 100 of Biofeedback Systems Ltd with the setting at mode one. This gives a click feedback, the click rate being proportional to the integrated EMG level shown on the meter. After the electrodes were in place the patient was asked to relax as much as possible the painful shoulder or lumbo-sacral region. This reduced the click rate considerably, but did not alter the pain of the affected part. The patient was then needled in the appropriate part of the hand or foot and again asked to relax the affected part as much as possible. In many instances the pain in the shoulder or lumbo-sacral area disappeared, and the patient if previously unable to touch his toes was then able to do so. The click rate though remained the same (as when the patient consciously relaxed) as did the meter reading. If the clicking was turned off for the duration of the experiment, and the instrument turned in such a way so that the patient could not see the silent meter, the result was the same.

Conclusions

All of the above experiments, were in the nature of a pilot trial. If the pilot trial had been successful the experiments would have continued and involved a larger number of patients.

This, of course, means that each of the experiments was performed only a limited number of times. It is just conceivable, if we had persisted with the experiments, a positive result would have ensued. It is also possible, if we had tried the above experiments in many different ways, we could in the end have demonstrated a positive result.

My main purpose in publishing these experiments, most of which were carried out many years ago and nearly forgotten, is to show that research into acupuncture is far from simple. Many articles have been published in specialist acupuncture journals and also general medical journals, in which the conclusions drawn are opposed to the ones in this chapter.

As acupuncture helps a reasonable proportion of patients with the appropriate type of disease, it should be possible to demonstrate in some objective manner, the effect of treating a patient. The hopefully objective research which several colleagues and I have performed has had no positive result. In the same way, when I have investigated in sufficient detail some of the claims of others, their results could quite possibly be reinterpreted as also negative.

Obviously a considerably greater effort is required. Perhaps if the amount of time, thought and effort which is applied to western medicine, is likewise applied to acupuncture, it will bear fruit. Many doctors and researchers experience difficulty in separating traditional acupuncture, from what *actually happens*: a deficiency which I hope is clarified by this book.

The Mind Versus the Body, or the Mind Plus the Body

At present I believe there are certain aspects of acupuncture which are purely physical: the effect of needling a joint locally seems to be similar to that of a local steroid injection.

Other aspects of acupuncture are probably largely psychosomatic. In this respect it is similar to a reasonable proportion of general practice.

I think quite a substantial part of the success of acupuncture lies somewhere between the mental and the physical aspects: if there is only the mental treatment it does not help; if there is only physical treatment it likewise fails.

Many patients who have headaches or migraine, are treated by doctors practising acupuncture as a reasonable proportion of them are helped by acupuncture, even though they may have had their symptoms for ten, twenty or thirty years. An acupuncture point frequently employed for this purpose is liver 3 (between the 1st and 2nd metatarsals) or bladder 62 (below the lateral malleolus). On several occasions I have needled the ends of toes or the sole of the foot, in a random manner, in positions where there are no acupuncture points – and yet the patient's headache or migraine improved, (though this has not been done often enough to know if the same proportion of patients are helped). Yet patients who stub their toes against a rock or who walk for a few moments with a stone in their shoe, experiencing just as much pain as if they had been needled, have no relief of their headache or migraine.

Conversely a psychiatrist is mostly of less benefit in headache or migraine than a doctor practising acupuncture.

It is this peculiar combination of the physical stimulus of a needle prick, together with psychological factors, which seems to produce the results one sees in acupuncture. This is of course a largely new concept in medicine, a concept which should be considered when designing research projects. A rose is a physical object, but a *beautiful* rose is a nonscientific concept as it is a combination of something physical and non-physical. 'Man does not live by bread alone. . . .'

All Roads Lead to Rome

Acupuncture encompasses several phenomena and probably various mechanisms for:

1. On some occasions a needle prick anywhere on the body, is sufficient to produce relief of the patient's symptoms.
2. On other occasions the needle prick may be anywhere in the appropriate quarter of the body.
3. On still other occasions the stimulus has seemingly to be in the correct dermatome, myotome, sclerotome, vasculartome or other area of this magnitude of size.
4. On yet other occasions stimulation of a reflexly tender area, often the size of the palm of the hand, produces the best result. The tender areas mentioned by Kellgren in Chapter I Fig. 9 and in Chapter VI are of this nature.
5. If a trigger point, perhaps a centimetre in diameter can be found, and it is needled, not infrequently the best result ensues.

Often, but by no means always, needling a trigger point of a tender area is more effective than needling anywhere on the body or even in the correct dermatome. If a trigger point or tender area are hypersensitive, or in a 'strong reactor' (see Chapter IV), local needling may aggravate the condition, and hence treatment of a distant area is more appropriate.

Trigger points, or reflexly tender areas are not necessarily relevant to the disease in question. Patients with a painful shoulder not infrequently have a tender area, about two centimetres in diameter, at the insertion of the deltoid, halfway down the lateral side of the humerus. Needling this tender area has no effect.

All Roads Emanate from Rome

The reverse of all the above phenomena may also be observed in at least a limited number of patients:

1. If a patient has, say, a mild pain in the neck, it may be alleviated by needling the appropriate place in the foot (say, liver 3, between the 1st and 2nd metatarsals).
2. If a patient has mild lumbago, it may also be relieved by needling liver 3.
3. If a patient has mild pain in the neck, headache, lumbago and nausea; all four symptoms may likewise benefit when liver 3 is needled. This relief may occur a few seconds after stimulation, thus excluding humoral factors, for the blood or lymphatic flow would be too slow to conduct a chemical substance from one part of the body to another in this short time.

Sensitized Segments of the Cord

One of the few possible explanations for this phenomenon, which I have discussed with the neurologist Peter Nathan, is as follows:

1. If one has a pain in the neck the appropriate part of the cervical cord is sensitized. If one has lumbago certain sections of the lower lumbar or upper sacral cord are sensitized.
2. If a specific part of the skin is needled, the stimulus has a tendency to spread to the rest of the body. This has been shown experimentally by:

   a. Sato and Schmidt (Chapter V) who demonstrated that a stimulus had a primary immediate effect in the same and adjacent segments, and also a delayed general sympathetic response over the whole body mediated by the sympathetic centre in the medulla.

   b. Le Bars, Dickenson and Besson (Chapter XI) have shown that stimulation, nearly anywhere, will inhibit the appreciation of pain in nearly every other part of the body. This is mediated by convergent dorsal neurones, which receive both a noxious and non-noxious input.

Thus a stimulus, applied anywhere in the body, probably often spreads throughout all segments via the above two and probably other means. When this stimulus reaches a sensitized area (such as the neck or lumbar area in our example) it has an effect and hence reduces the pain or muscle spasm. A nonsensitized part of the cord is not influenced, according to this theory, and hence is uninfluenced by the relatively gentle stimulus of ordinary acupuncture.

IX

RADIATION AND REFERRED SENSATION OR PAIN

It is frequently possible, when needling a patient, to obtain radiation or a referred mild pain or sensation. This is most likely to happen if the periosteum is stimulated and more particularly so in certain positions such as the region of the sacro-iliac joint. This phenomenon is less likely to occur if the skin, subcutaneous tissues or muscles are needled.

This radiation is quite different from the sudden, shooting, severe and rapidly moving pain one has if a major nerve trunk is needled or the ulnar nerve is compressed at the elbow.

The radiation sensation is usually gentle and may take several seconds to traverse the length of a limb. It may be so gentle that one is only aware of it when sitting comfortably, without distraction, in relaxed surroundings; the effect being like a gentle breeze blowing on one's foot, or a slight tingling sensation. Usually it is experienced as a mild pain travelling a variable distance along a path a few millimetres to a centimetre wide.

Sometimes the radiation or referred sensation, may start from the site of the needle prick. Sometimes it may only be felt at a distant site. Sometimes it may emanate from the needle prick, travel along a more or less straight course all the way to a distant site. Sometimes en route to the distant site, certain sections of the 'path' may be missing. Sometimes in a distant site it may, particularly in the head, neck and shoulders, produce a feeling of warmth; or if referred to the nose a 'crackling'.

If the region of the sacro-iliac joint is needled and a patient has pain at the back of the thigh, the radiation will most frequently go to the back of the thigh. If instead the patient had pain on the medial side of the thigh and *exactly the same region of the sacro-iliac joint is needled,* the radiation sensation or pain will travel to the medial side of the thigh. If the pain was on the lateral side of the thigh and again the same region of the sacro-iliac joint is needled, the needle pain will radiate to the lateral side of the thigh, in the majority of instances. Likewise with the anterior of the thigh.

It is thus apparent that if a certain specific area of periosteum is needled and a patient has radiation within the possibilities of referred pain from the needled area, the radiation will then go to the patient's painful area.

The course of the radiation, does not follow the path of a major nerve, artery, vein, bone or meridian. This phenomenon of radiation, perhaps gave the ancient Chinese their original conception of meridians, except that if one observes carefully, the pathway of the radiation and its destination, are seen to be infinitely variable. Amongst the infinitely variable possibilities of radiation and its destination there are perhaps, but only perhaps, certain preferred paths which on balance seem to be travelled more frequently than others. But even these preferred paths do not correspond with any obvious anatomical structure or even the meridians.

Radiation may be used clinically in acupuncture. If for example a patient has pain in the thumb, it may be treated, if it is an easily reversible condition, by needling the periosteum of the radius, anywhere along its whole length so as to elicit a radiation of pain into the thumb. If exactly the same place on the radius is needled, but without radiation to the thumb, the treatment may well give ease, but it is less likely to be successful than if there were radiation into the thumb.

If the upper third of the tibialis anterior is needled so that the needle goes through to the periosteum of the lateral side of the tibia (see Fig. 21), there may be radiation down the front of the shin, the front of the ankle and into the toes. If a patient has pain of a mild, easily reversible nature in the ankle, radiation to the ankle may alleviate the condition. If the pain is instead in the transverse arch of the foot radiation has to reach as far as the transverse arch for the most likely optional effect.

In the case of pain in the ankle, it is unlikely (but occasionally possible), for the radiation from the tibialis anterior to go below the ankle, into the transverse arch or toes. It seems as if the site of pain is often the 'end station'. If the pain is in the toes, the radiation is more likely to reach the toes, than if the pain were in the ankle.

It is considerably easier to obtain radiation in a 'strong reactor' (see Chapter IV) than in a normal reactor. Radiation may go from one end of the body to another in a strong reactor, whilst in a normal or slow reactor the distance travelled by the radiation is nearly always less or even considerably less. Sometimes in normal or slow reactors, one has to manipulate the needle for a long time before obtaining radiation, whilst in a strong reactor radiation may occur in the first few seconds.

On a few occasions I have deliberately tried to needle, with a thin acupuncture needle, a major nerve trunk, to obtain the shooting pain well known from compression of the ulnar nerve at the elbow. Interestingly it was much easier to elicit this shooting pain in a strong reactor. Presumably the diameter of the same nerve is the same in a strong and slow reactor. Perhaps the threshold of stimulation is lower in a strong reactor?

It is easier to achieve radiation in the limbs, than in most positions on the trunk and the radiation travels more often centrifugally than centripetally.

Various Chinese authors have stated that inflation of a blood pressure cuff across the path of the radiation, stops the radiation at the level of the inflated cuff. On some occasions I have merely pinched the skin in one place along the path of the radiation, which stopped the radiation going beyond the pinched area.

X

REFLEXES ELICITED BY STRONG STIMULATION

Relevant research has recently been conducted at Goteborg.*
Cholera toxin was placed in the lumen of the jejunum in anaesthe-
tised rats, which produced a large secretion of fluid into the lumen
of the isolated segment of jejunum.

The sciatic nerve was stimulated for 60 minutes, at some 10
times twitch threshold, at 3 Hertz, with a duration of 0.2 milliseconds. The intestinal fluid secretion was considerably reduced in
most rats, for 30 minutes after stimulation had ceased. Thereafter
intestinal secretion slowly returned to normal values.

In a further series of experiments, the sciatic nerve was stimulated in rats whose jejunum had not been subjected to cholera
toxin. In these experiments the intestinal secretion was largely
unaffected.

In another group of rats the tissue surrounding the superior mesenteric artery and vein was divided, thus depriving the jejunum of
its extrinsic autonomic innervation. The jejunum subsequently had
cholera toxin placed in the lumen, which as previously increased
secretion of fluid. Sciatic stimulation did not influence jejunal
secretion in this group, thus demonstrating the importance of the
intestinal innervation.

It is interesting to note that sciatic stimulation had an effect only
in the rats with a diseased jejunum and not in those who did not

*Cassuto, J., Larssen, P., Yao, T., Jodal, M., Thorén, P., Andersson, S., Lund-
gren, O. The effect of stimulating somatic afferents on cholera secretion in the rat
small intestine. Acta Physiologica Scandinavica, 1982, 116: 443–446.

have cholera toxin. This corresponds with the clinical experience of acupuncture: it is possible to affect a region of the body which is not functioning correctly, but it is extremely difficult to alter the function of a region which is completely normal.

It should be noted that the above-mentioned stimulation was continued for an hour (it had less effect when tried for only 30 minutes), whilst one usually only stimulates for a few seconds in acupuncture. Normally by acupuncture, one only treats easily reversible physiological processes. Perhaps the scope of acupuncture could be increased to treat more severe conditions, using long continued stimulation.

The same laboratory* has used the same method of sciatic nerve stimulation in unanaesthetised, spontaneously hypertensive rats. They found that during a 30 minute period of sciatic nerve stimulation: the blood pressure, the heart rate and splanchnic nerve activity remained the same, or even increased. Thereafter, possibly after a delay of one or two hours: the blood pressure was reduced (from 160 mmHg to 140 mmHg), there was reduced splanchnic nerve activity, and mild bradycardia. Interestingly these depressive effects could last up to 12 hours.

All the experiments mentioned in this chapter required a longer period of stimulation and stronger stimulation than is usual in therapeutic acupuncture. It thus resembles the type of stimulation used in acupuncture analgesia.

---

*Yao, T., Andersson, S., Thorén, P. Long lasting cardiovascular depression induced by acupuncture-like stimulation of the sciatic nerve in unanaesthetised hypertensive rats. Brain Research, 1982: 240, 77–85.

XI

DIFFUSE NOXIOUS INHIBITORY CONTROL

by ANTHONY DICKENSON

An underlying principle of acupuncture is the relief or alleviation of pain somewhere in the body by application of a peripheral stimulus either by needling or electro-acupuncture. In investigating the electro-physiological basis for acupuncture the first criterion is to record the activity of a class of neurone which plays a role in the processes leading to the sensation of pain. It is impossible to extra-polate from neuronal activities to pain sensation but neurones responding to noxious stimuli can be presumed to be involved, to some extent, in nociception. Pain arising from the activation of nociceptors in the skin, muscles, viscera, etc. is transmitted by fine calibre peripheral fibres, the C fibres, which make contact with neurones located in the spinal cord or trigeminal complex. These central neurones responding to noxious inputs fall into two distinct classes. One type of neurone, responding only to noxious pinch and heat, is located in lamina 1 in the superficial layer of the dorsal part of the spinal cord. Despite this selective response to noxious pinch and heat, as most of these neurones extend for only 2–3 seg-ments and do not project up to the brain, and as none responds to muscular or visceral pain, it is unlikely that this class of cell is involved in pain in clinical practice which is rarely from skin origins.

Deeper in the dorsal horn, in lamina 5, another class of neurone can be found, which due to the variety of inputs arriving at the cell body has been designated as a convergent neurone. These cells respond to inputs from the skin, muscles and viscera; many of them project to higher centres of the brain, and the neurones respond in a sustained and powerful manner to noxious heat and pinch. However the cells additionally respond to innocuous peripheral stimuli.

There are two types of peripheral stimuli, both relevant to acupuncture-like procedures, which inhibit the activities of these convergent neurones and which may explain the analgesic effects of these procedures. The independence of these controls suggest that there may be two different bases for acupuncture. The first inhibitory control on these cells is the so called segmental inhibition. Surrounding the excitatory receptive field of these cells, the area of the periphery from which the cells can be activated, is a zone inside which light tactile stimuli can inhibit the pain related activities of these cells. Similarly, electrical activation of the touch fibres can block the activity of these cells. The segmental nature of these controls is critical in that the conditioning stimuli must be applied locally and so acupuncture acting from distant areas of the body must be doing so by a different mechanism. The clinical use of low intensity peripheral stimulation applied locally and known as transcutaneous nerve stimulation (TNS) is derived from these segmental inhibitory effects. So what then is the mechanism of acupuncture effects produced from distant areas of the body and of the acupuncture relief of pain using higher intensities of peripheral stimulation?

Recent electrophysiological studies by Le Bars, Dickenson and Besson seem to provide a basis for the stronger forms of acupuncture acting from far-flung areas of the body. They have found that every convergent neurone either in the spinal cord or the facial equivalent, the trigeminal complex, can be powerfully, and in some cases, completely inhibited by a strong stimulus applied elsewhere on the body. Thus, a convergent neurone with an input from the hindpaw of the animal can be excited by noxious pinch, noxious heat and light touch or electrical stimulation of the incoming peripheral fibres emanating from the defined receptive field of the neurone. If the neurone is steadily activated by one of these inputs, mimicking the state of the neurone in a condition of pain in humans, a strong stimulus applied to the tail, forepaws, ears, nose or elsewhere on the body will inhibit the response of the neurone.

The conditioning stimulus must be at or above the pain threshold and can be natural (mechanical or thermal) chemical or electrical. The inhibitions, so produced, have been described as diffuse noxious inhibitory controls (DNIC) because of their nature. They rely on complex neural loops passing up from the spinal cord and down again from the brain to produce their final effects in the spinal cord. Certain of the neurones modulated by these effects are neurones which project up to the brain via the spinothalmic, the spinoreticular and other tracts, and so their inhibitions can be presumed to alter the quality of the pain sensation. DNIC produce powerful and long-lasting inhibitions of all activities of these neurones whilst other classes of neurones are not influenced. These inhibitions in general outlast the period of application of the peripheral stimulus by several fold and these prolonged post-effects may go towards explaining the long duration of pain relief following acupuncture-like stimulation. But the maximal inhibition still only lasts for four minutes.

Within the limitations of electrophysiological approaches (in that there is the inherent assumption that the activity of neurones represents a functional role) these results demonstrate that both a local and a distant (unrelated either in terms of dermatomes or segments) stimulus can reduce the activity of nociceptive neurones. The local effects seem to depend on innocuous afferent impulses whilst the distant seem to be via high threshold or noxious afferents.

There is now ample clinical and behavioural evidence to support these electrophysiological findings. Early work, originating in the thirties, has amply illustrated the ability of a noxious input to one area of the body to influence the sensation of pain arising from another region. This phenomenon has been illustrated by use of both thermally and mechanically induced pain. In a recent review of the clinical use of peripheral stimulation to reduce the intensity of pain, Andersson has concluded that there are distinct differences, both in terms of causes and effects, between local and distant pain relieving procedures.

The local or segmental mechanisms require low intensity and high frequency stimuli and underlie transcutaneous nerve stimulation (TNS) as used clinically. However, acupuncture-like stimuli require higher intensity and low frequency stimuli and according

to Andersson afford a greater relief of pain in terms of both duration and degree of the analgesia.

These conclusions accord well with the neurophysiological evidence for two separate routes of action of peripheral pain relieving
stimuli. The distant diffuse acupuncture effects use more complex
neural and chemical pathways. This indicates that there are many
potentially effective means of influencing pain by tapping into
these systems and may explain why attitudes, environment and
other psychological variables can interact with acupuncture and
pain.

References

Nathan, P. W. The gate control theory of pain. A critical review. Brain, 1976, 99: 123–
    158.
Le Bars, D., Dickenson, A. & Besson, J. M. Diffuse Noxious Inhibitory Controls
    (DNIC). I. Effects on dorsal horn convergent neurones in the rat. Pain, 1979, 6:
    283–304.
Le Bars, D., Dickenson, A. & Besson, J. M. Diffuse Noxious Inhibitory Controls
    (DNIC). II. Lack of effect on non-convergent neurones, supraspinal involvement
    and theoretical implications. Pain, 1979, 6: 305–327.
Andersson, S. A. Pain control by sensory stimulation. Advances in Pain Research and
    Therapy, Vol. 3, Raven Press, New York, 1979.
Melzack, R. Prolonged relief of pain by brief, intense transcutaneous somatic stimu-
    lation. Pain, 1975, 1: 357–373.
Chung, S. H. & Dickenson, A. H. Pain, enkephalin and acupuncture. Nature, 1980,
    283–344.
Berlin, S. A., Goodell, B. S. & Wolff, H. G. Studies on pain. A.M.A. Arch. Neurol.,
    1958, 80: 533–543.

XII

ACUPUNCTURE ANALGESIA: AN ELUSIVE ENIGMA

Acupuncture was virtually unknown, except in the Far East, before 1971. A small number of doctors were practising therapeutic acupuncture in Europe and Russia; the former had learnt it indirectly via 'colonial' trade, the latter as they were 'fraternal' neighbours.

Most of the doctors practising acupuncture, myself included, were considered part of the lunatic fringe: largely good-natured dreamers, who fooled themselves as much as their patients. We were regarded more as a joke than a pestilence. At that time I gave a certain number of talks at the monthly meetings of local medical societies. Normally these were serious meetings discussing such important topics as surgery of the prostate. Once a year though, there was a ladies' meeting, and it was on this occasion that I gave a lecture—instead of I suppose, a film of Donald Duck.

This was all changed overnight by President Nixon of the United States, who as far as I know was not the slightest bit interested in acupuncture. Unwittingly he transported acupuncture to the West, much as a man may unwittingly carry a flea from one country to another. As far as we are concerned he is the patron saint of acupuncture.

Prior to 1971 there was virtually no contact between the U.S.A. and China. In that year President Nixon inaugurated the 'open doors' policy with China and visited that country. The well-known and respected journalist James Reston went to China at about the same time, had appendicitis which was operated on in China in the normal way with chemical anaesthesia. Postoperatively he had, as is not unusual, some pain which was treated by acupuncture. This was all correctly described by James Reston in a long article in the New York Times and from there spread to the newspapers of the world. I have met many people who read this article with enthusiasm, but somehow they misread it, thinking that the acupuncture had been used for anaesthesia, instead of what was probably only wind pain: the spread of acupuncture to the West was largely brought about by hot air!

At the same time news reached the West that acupuncture was being used in China as an anaesthetic for operations ranging from tonsillectomy to open heart surgery. Most of us in the West, who had been practising acupuncture for several years were surprised, as I doubt if any of us had noticed a patient becoming anaethetised whilst we were treating them for migraine, lumbago or anything else. If one of us had a minor ailment which we had treated ourselves by acupuncture, there was likewise no anaesthesia.

In the early 1960s a comprehensive textbook of acupuncture was published in China which described acupuncture anaethesia for tonsillectomy. After reading all the details carefully I tried this. There was either no anaethesia at all, or so little that it was difficult to recognise.

Then in 1971 the Nixon–Reston bombshell hit us. The acupuncture doctors in the West tried furiously to imitate the 'success' the Chinese had with acupuncture anaethesia. We thought we had been delinquent pupils of acupuncture, the swine who had not noticed the pearls. Some doctors in the West had spectacular success with acupuncture anaesthesia and wrote textbooks on the subject up to 1000 pages long, gave courses on the technique and thought they would make their colleagues the anaesthetists bankrupt. Some anaethetists thought it was 'better to join them than fight them' and the membership of various acupuncture societies increased astronomically.

The early 1970s were the 'boom years' of acupuncture. It was a time when many did not realise there was a difference between therapeutic acupuncture and the fairy tale world of acupuncture anaesthesia. I remember on one occasion Pan American Airways telephoned to say a Boeing 747 had just arrived at Heathrow, full of American tourists. They all wished to experience acupuncture— and would I treat them (in those days there were virtually no acupuncturists in the U.S.A. outside Chinatown). I wished they had telephoned when I started my practice in 1959. Doctors were so keen to learn the miracle from the East that on occasion one week courses were run, attended by 500 doctors at a time. I was treated as an important personality, something that never happened before, or since. I was seated next to astronauts; gave lectures over the whole world; and was honoured to be met at the airport by a young Californian doctor wearing a suit—he had never owned a suit before.

At the same time somewhat more serious investigation of acupuncture anaesthesia was taking place:

Initially I tried to anaesthetise a friend in the tonsillar area, using the technique described at that time in the Chinese literature, by stimulating Li4 (between the 1st and 2nd metacarpals) and S44 (just proximial to the web between the 2nd and 3rd toes). It had no effect. Later I repeated the procedure and afterwards, by chance, pricked the tonsillar area with a needle. With incredulous surprise my friend realised she felt no pain from the pin prick. She could feel the needle going through the flesh. If she moved her tongue round her mouth or if I put my finger in the tonsillar area it felt normal. Temperature sense was likewise normal and the appearance was normal. Hence it was obvious that only pain was affected, no other sensation. Henceforth it was called acupuncture analgesia, not acupuncture anaesthesia, something I think the Chinese had not clarified at that time. I do not think this result was psychological, as the first attempt had failed. In addition my friend and I (due to the vague Chinese descriptions available to us) had expected a sensation similar to a dental nerve block, in which there is absence of all sensation (analgesia) and an unpleasant swollen feeling.

The surprise about this experiment, confirmed by later experiments, was that neither the patient nor the doctor knows if there is analgesia; or if it is present, where it is. To discover if there is analgesia one must prick the patient from head to toe noting if there are, or are not, any areas of partial or complete analgesia.

A simple technique is to use a 23-gauge hypodermic needle. The pricking should be done with equal force over the whole body, or at least that part of the body under consideration. In my experience the pricks should be firm enough to draw a little blood with say half the pricks. If the pricks are too light the result can be confusing.

In 1971 and 1972 I tried acupuncture analgesia 100 times in 35 friends and patients, which were later published in detail.* In essence the results were rather mediocre, and at the same time difficult to interpret.

In the best group of patients there was a relatively uniform analgesia over a specified area. But even within this analgesic area a certain number of pin pricks revealed normal sensation of pain. There was never the complete analgesia one has with a well-given local anaesthetic. In 1972 I considered that some 10% of patients belonged to this rather badly defined 'best' group. Later I thought I had been too enthusiastic and would now rather suggest 5%.

I investigated with the physiologist Tim Horder two patients who belonged to this best group. We knew (though the patients did not), that if acupuncture point T5, on the posterior aspect of the forearm, is stimulated, there may be analgesia in the ipsilateral chest wall, both anteriorly and posteriorly. We told the patients though that the opposite forearm to the one being needled would become analgesic. When the experiment was then finally performed, both patients noticed that there was no analgesia where they had been told to expect it (the contralateral forearm), but that analgesia was present in the correct area (the ipsilateral chest wall).

The above experiment and also the unexpected discovery of analgesia in the tonsillar area mentioned previously, suggests that at least part of the mechanism of acupuncture analgesia is physiological. This of course does not exclude a psychological factor in addition. Nor does it clarify whether the physiological or psychological factor is dominant.

It was found that the 5% or so of patients who respond well to acupuncture analgesia are the 'strong reactors' mentioned in Chapter IV. In therapeutic acupuncture more than 5% of the population are strong reactors. Acupuncture analgesia is effective among only the best of the strong reactors and hence these patients might be called 'hyper-strong reactors'.

Apart from the 5% hyper-strong reactors, there is a variable proportion of people who have a mild or very mild degree of analgesia. This milder analgesia is usually patchy: rather like the Aegean Sea

---

*Mann, F. B. Acupuncture Analgesia. British Journal of Anasthesia, 1974, 46: 361–4.

studded with islands. In the better patients the analgesia corresponds to the all-enveloping sea; whilst in the less responsive
patients the analgesia merely corresponds to the small islands.

Acupuncture analgesia is an interesting neurophysiological
phenomenon occurring in hyper-strong reactors. It is of little practical use however. It cannot be completely forgotten, as it does
exist—but only just. Whether it could ever be further developed is,
I think, rather open to doubt. A surprisingly large number of
doctors who practise acupuncture disagree with my rather negative
attitude to acupuncture analgesia. Some say the effects are better,
some even say the effects are very much better.

Some anaesthetists combine chemical anaesthesia with acupuncture anaesthesia, particularly in frail, elderly, rather ill patients who
supposedly might have difficulty in withstanding only normal
anaesthetics (although this group of patients require less anaesthetic
agents anyway). They are usually given normal premedication,
and a 50–50 mixture of gas and oxygen. Electro-acupuncture anaesthesia is done in addition.

Other anaesthetists do the same as the above, but in addition
curarise and intubate their patients. In this curarised state they are
able to pass much larger currents through the acupuncture needles
or electrodes, and hence supposedly the acupuncture has a stronger
effect. This would not be possible in a non-curarised patient as his
muscles would go into tetanic spasm with a current of this magnitude.

The anaesthetists who use the above techniques think they use
only about a third of the dose of chemical agents they would use
under normal circumstances. I have discussed this with other
anaesthetists, who say that if an anaesthetist is particularly
interested in using minimal doses of anaesthesic he is usually able to
do so, and particularly in frail, elderly and ill patients. These anaesthetists think the acupuncture contributes very little or nothing to
the overall anaesthesia.

Once again, however, the process is tedious, and probably even
if it works, is not often a practical proposition. An expert, whether
in the Far East or the West, can quite often demonstrate anaesthesia, as he knows how to select the hyper-strong reactor.